Cooking with
Superfoods

h.f.ullmann

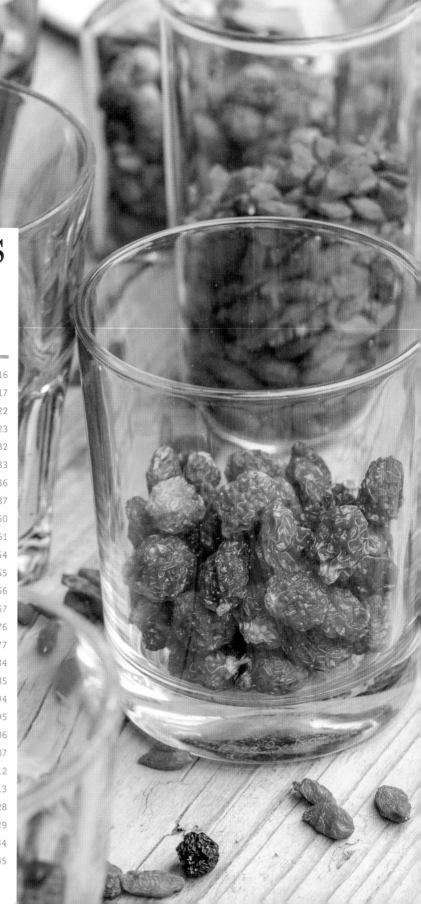

CONTENTS

SUPERFOOD PROFILES

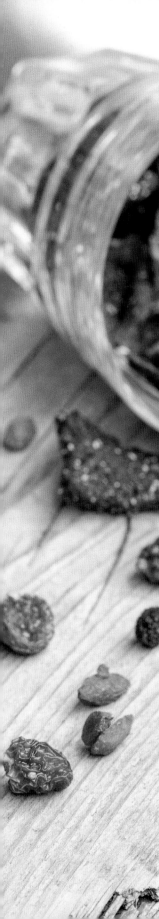

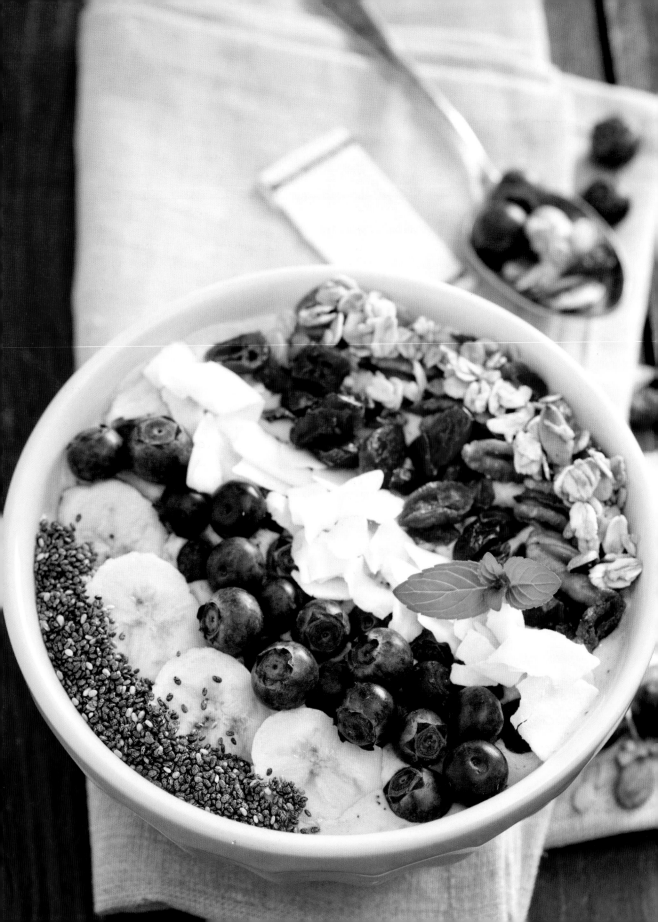

WHAT ARE SUPERFOODS?

"Superfoods," a name coined in the United States and used as far back as the early 20th century, have become popular, however, only in recent years. The term first appeared in the *Oxford Dictionary* back in 1915, when a super-food was defined as "a nutrient-rich food considered to be especially beneficial for health and well-being and preventive against diseases." In fact, by their very nature as (mainly) plant-based foods, superfoods contain particularly high amounts of vitamins, minerals, trace elements, dietary fiber, phytochemicals, and antioxidants. This means that they have above-average high nutrient density, which is used to determine the quality of a particular foodstuff. "Nutrient density" describes the ratio of essential nutrients such as vitamins, minerals, and phytochemicals to the calorie content. So food that contains a high nutrient density provides a lot of nutrients and at the same time has low energy content. Our energy requirements in today's more sedentary society have reduced, while at the same time the amount of nutrients we need remains the same. This means that foodstuffs with a high nutrient density are especially important for a modern, healthy diet. Fruit, vegetables, pulses, whole wheat and whole milk products, and lean meat and fish all have an extra-high nutrient density. The list is headed by plant-based "superfoods" with their extraordinarily rich nutrient density.

Everyone benefits from superfoods, irrespective of his or her state of health, eating habits, or age. Whether you are a meat-eater, flexitarian, vegetarian, or vegan, you would do well to include high-grade food in your diet. During certain phases of life, eating superfoods makes particular sense: Pregnant women, young mothers, children, athletes, and the elderly all gain advantage from an extra-healthy diet. But superfoods also give us an energy boost whenever our energy levels are drained, whether we are recovering from an illness or during stressful times in our lives. Superfoods have many preventive effects on our health (see pp. 7–8).

Superfoods can be added to some baked goods to make them a source of health-giving nutrients.

NUTRITIONAL INFORMATION

All the recipes in this book are designed for two people. The nutritional tables show the quantities per portion, i.e. half of the total amount, unless otherwise indicated.

THE ORAC VALUE

Apart from the nutrient density (p. 5), what exactly makes a particular food a super-food? Another factor in the definition is what is known as the ORAC (Oxygen Radical Absorbance Capacity) value. This represents the concentration levels of antioxidants in foodstuffs: The higher the ORAC value, and hence antioxidant content, the healthier the particular food item is said to be. Here is a brief overview of the ORAC values of some superfoods for comparison:

Food	Av. ORAC value (µmol TE/3½ oz or 100 g)
Avocado	1,933
Blueberries, fresh	6,552
Broccoli, cooked	1,552
Broccoli, raw	3,083
Cocoa powder, raw	80,933
Cranberries, raw	9,584
Dates (Medjool), fresh	2,387
Ginger, fresh	14,840
Ginger, ground	29,041
Spinach, raw	1,515
Sprouts (radishes)	2,184
Walnuts	13,541

Source: U.S. Department of Agriculture, 2010

Superfoods in dried or powder form, such as acai powder, ground ginger, or cocoa powder, usually have a far higher ORAC value than fresh foods like spinach or avocado. In these cases, the nutrients are in a compressed form, but we consume them only in small amounts, unlike the fresh foods we eat in far larger quantities. The ORAC value can also vary depending on the cultivar, harvesting time, and state of ripeness. A plant-based food protects itself against the sun's UV rays with antioxidants: During its growth phase, the longer it is exposed to sunlight, the more antioxidants it contains. In tests, organically grown food has come out better, containing more antioxidants than conventionally grown fruits and vegetables. The results of a study by the University of California, Davis conducted over a ten-year period showed that organic tomatoes, for example, contained twice as many flavonoids (p. 9) as traditionally grown ones.

The recommended daily amount of ORAC values in food varies: Many nutritionists now work on the assumption that we can protect our bodies from harmful free radicals with a daily intake of 5,000 to 7,000 µmol TE / 3½ oz or 100 g. To give an example, 7,000 ORAC units correspond roughly to just over 3½ oz (100 g) of blueberries or around ½ cup (52 g) of walnuts. The exact amount of superfoods required depends on an individual's particular lifestyle: A city dweller constantly exposed to noise and doing a stressful job, for instance, needs more nutrients than a rural resident with a quiet occupation. The ORAC value is however an in vitro laboratory result, not one that is produced in the human body. The extent to which the ORAC values can be applied to the human body is still scientifically inconclusive.

ANTIOXIDANTS AND FREE RADICALS

The human body produces what are known as "free radicals" during metabolism. They are fundamentally useful in supporting the immune system and maintaining good health—as long as they do not become too numerous. Then their positive effect is reversed: So the quantity of free radicals determines whether they are beneficial or harmful. Various factors can result in free radicals gaining the upper hand in our bodies—an unhealthy, unvarying diet; stress; anxiety; environmental influences like UV rays, emissions, pesticides, and chemicals; lack of sleep; medication; alcohol, cigarettes, and drugs; even extreme sport. The "oxidative stress" associated with excessive free radicals can eventually result in our cells being attacked and the DNA damaged. This is believed to be a causal factor in the aging process and life expectancy. Free radicals are also suspected of causing a wide range of diseases such as cancer, arteriosclerosis, arthritis, diabetes, and Alzheimer's.

Antioxidants are effective against free radicals, hence their description as "free radical scavengers." Our own body's defense system can also produce antioxidants, protecting us from oxidative stress and cell damage. In addition, we obtain highly effective antioxidants from natural foodstuffs. As these important protective agents are particularly prevalent in superfoods, they play a key role in our immune system and overall health. By contrast, several studies have shown that taking high doses of artificially produced vitamins and antioxidants has no, or even adverse, effects on our health. The motto "More is better!" has turned out to be completely false in the case of the "super-pills" widely used in the United States. On the other hand, we can effectively protect our health with natural nutrients, through a varied diet containing mainly plant-based foods that includes superfoods.

SOURCES OF ANTIOXIDANTS

These protective substances are found mainly in different types of fruits and vegetables, berries, herbs, edible wild plants, nuts, seeds, and fish. Vitamins A, C, and E are classed as antioxidants, as are secondary plant substances like carotenoids (beta-carotene) and the large group of polyphenols including anthocyanins and flavonoids.

VITAMINS

The vitamins with antioxidant properties are A, C, and E. Particularly large amounts of **vitamin C** are found in goji berries (p. 17), broccoli (p. 85), kale (p. 106), spinach (p. 76), blackcurrants, lemons (p. 95), and wild berries such as rosehips and sea buckthorn. Vitamin C is an effective antioxidant against free radicals. It stimulates the immune system and strengthens connective tissue, bones, blood vessels, and teeth. The body needs this vitamin for a whole range of metabolic processes, including the release of hormones. Vitamin C also promotes the absorption of iron and calcium in the intestines. Another "cell protector" is **vitamin E**: It is found mainly in vegetable oils like flaxseed oil (p. 67), wheat germ oil, and sunflower oil. High levels of vitamin E are also present, however, in fat-rich foods like avocados (p. 51), nuts (walnuts, p. 112), and seeds (hemp seeds, p. 55; chia seeds, p. 16), and in fish like salmon, mackerel, and herring. Vitamin E is also an antioxidant that protects our body cells. It is believed to counteract deposits in blood vessels and inhibit blood clotting, and thus plays a role in the prevention of thromboses, heart attacks, arteriosclerosis, and strokes. It is also important in fat metabolism, and good for healthy skin and hair. For **vitamin A**, see beta-carotene.

SECONDARY PLANT SUBSTANCES

Secondary plant substances are classified into different groups according to their chemical structure and their function for plants: Just some of the many examples are carotenoids, flavonoids, anthocyanins, sulfides, phytosterols, and phenol acids. Thousands of different secondary plant substances have been discovered in our food. They have a whole range of functions and a different composition in each plant-based food. While the role of primary substances (carbohydrates, proteins, and fats) in plants is to build and maintain them, the secondary plant substances are equally important. They too carry out vital functions: As agents that provide colors and flavors, they attract pollinators and seed spreaders, making them fundamental to propagation. They also act as protection against predators and pathogens, intense UV radiation, the harmful effects of climate, and free radicals. We incorporate this protection when we eat the plants.

Secondary plant substances are found in all types of fruits and vegetables, nuts, and seeds. These protective agents have a wide range of positive effects on our health. According to current research, they are believed to inhibit the development of cancer and cardiovascular disease, and protect us against arteriosclerosis, Alzheimer's, and various inflammatory conditions. They are assumed to have a positive effect on cholesterol levels, blood pressure, and blood sugar levels, and to help prevent blood clots. Secondary plant substances boost our resistance and can protect us from fungal, viral, and bacterial infections.

At the same time, organically grown plants usually contain higher levels of secondary plant substances than those grown traditionally—they are not treated with pesticides so they have to rely on using their own natural defense systems.

Carotenoids, which include over 600 known substances to date, form an important group of secondary plant substances. They use their light-filtering properties to protect the plants' leaves from the damaging effects of UV rays. They are believed to give humans a natural form of protection from the sun too, if enough carotenoids are introduced in the diet. **Beta-carotene** is one of the best known carotenoids, found mostly as the yellow/orange/red food coloring in pumpkins (p. 84), carrots, and goji berries (p. 17), and less visibly in blueberries (p. 33), broccoli (p. 85), spinach (p. 76), and kale (p. 106). After we have ingested it in food, our body converts beta-carotene into vitamin A. As an antioxidant, it protects us against oxidative stress (see p. 7). It is thought to reduce the risk of cancer and cardiovascular disease, and act as an anti-inflammatory. It is also important, among other things, for the immune system, skin, bone growth, and vision. Vitamin A plays a key role in retinal health, and this is why beta-carotene is often called the "eye vitamin."

Polyphenols are also classed as secondary plant substances and are found as coloring or flavoring agents in fruits and vegetables. They protect our body cells from the harmful effects of free radicals, and have cancer-inhibiting and anti-inflammatory properties. It is for this reason that including pomegranate in the diet is recommended by some organizations in cases of breast and prostate cancer. Polyphenols also provide protection against cardiovascular disease, as well as reducing fatty deposits in blood vessels and thus preventing arteriosclerosis. They are also believed to play a role in the prevention of Alzheimer's disease. Examples of foods with a particularly high polyphenol content include aronia berries (p. 23), pomegranates (p. 50), and raw cocoa (p. 128). The better-known polyphenols are **anthocyanins** and flavonoids. Anthocyanins give fruits and vegetables a dark red, purple-blue color, especially in the outer layers. They are found in large quantities in fruits like blueberries (p. 33), aronia berries (p. 23), cherries, acai berries (p. 36), red cabbage, and eggplant. **Flavonoids** are literally "little yellow things" (from the Latin *flavus*, "yellow") as they are often this color, though it is not always the case. Flavonoids give onions, bell peppers, and oranges their bright yellow to orange color, and are responsible for the red to purple color of beets, plums, and grapes. These plant substances are also found in nuts (walnuts, p. 112), kale (p. 106), broccoli (p. 85), and apples.

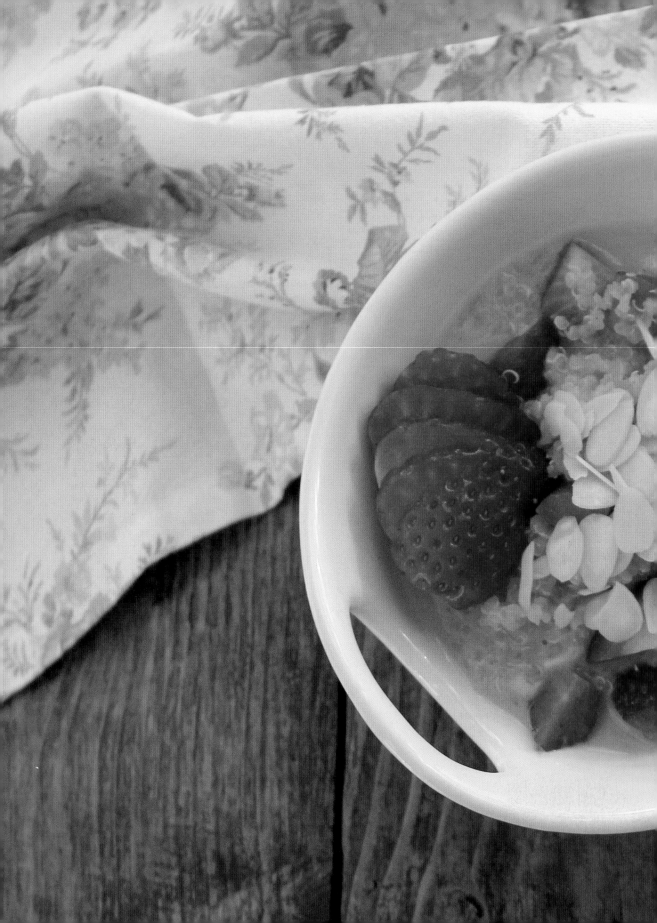

BREAKFAST

BREAD ROLLS WITH NUTS

AND BERRIES

MAKES 6–12
2 tbsp (18-20 g) shelled almonds
2 tbsp (15 g) shelled **walnuts**
1 cup (150 g) whole
wheat khorasan flour
⅔ cup (100 g) whole rye flour
½ sachet yeast (approx. 3 g)
1 tbsp (8 g) **chia seeds**
1 tbsp (8 g) sunflower seeds
⅓ cup (40 g) dried
unsweetened **cranberries**
salt

NUTRITIONAL VALUE

per roll (when making 9)

kcal	kJ	Protein	Fat	Carbo-hydrate
130	530	4	3	21

1. Coarsely chop the almonds and walnuts. Put them in a large bowl with the two flours, yeast, chia seeds, sunflower seeds, cranberries, and 1 cup (¼ liter) of lukewarm water. Knead with the dough attachment of a hand mixer and then mix in the salt.

2. Cover the dough and leave to prove for at least 30 minutes, or overnight.

3. Divide and shape the dough into 6 larger or 12 smaller rolls and place them on a cookie pan lined with wax paper. Bake in the oven at 475 °F/240 °C (not pre-heated) for about 20 minutes.

These little rolls go well with both sweet and savory toppings. You can also use other types of flour, for example 1⅔ cups (250 g) of whole spelt flour.

CHIA JAM

WITH BLACKBERRIES

MAKES approx. 1 cup (¼ liter)
7 oz (200 g) blackberries
2 tbsp (16 g) **chia seeds**

NUTRITIONAL VALUE

per 1 cup (¼ liter) jar

kcal	kJ	Protein	Fat	Carbo-hydrate
90	400	3	3	13

1. Pick over the blackberries, rinse briefly, drain, and whizz in a blender. Mix in the chia seeds with a spoon and leave the jam to soak in the refrigerator for at least 30 minutes.

You can make this "clean," sugar-free jam with any fruit you like. It keeps well for up to a week if stored in a sealed jar in the refrigerator. Optional: Add 1 tablespoon of agave syrup, honey, raw cane sugar, or coconut palm sugar.

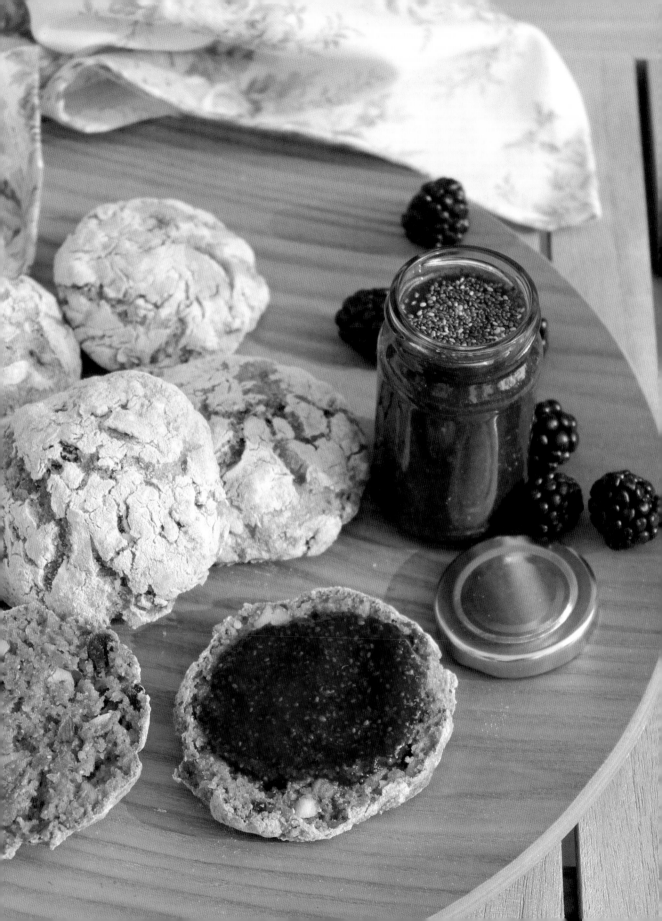

CHIA PUDDING
WITH MANGO AND COCONUT MILK

SERVES 2

1⅔ cups (400 ml) **coconut milk**
2 tbsp (16 g) **chia seeds**
1 mango
4 Cape gooseberries
1 tbsp (5 g) **shredded coconut** for garnish

NUTRITIONAL VALUE
per portion

kcal	kJ	Protein	Fat	Carbo-hydrate
120	480	2	3	20

1. Mix together the coconut milk and 1 tablespoon of chia seeds. Set to one side. Peel the mango, remove the pit, and coarsely chop the flesh. Remove the leaves from the Cape gooseberries.

2. Whizz the chopped mango, Cape gooseberries, 1 tablespoon of chia seeds, and 4 teaspoons (20 ml) of water in a blender. Divide the coconut mixture between two glasses or bowls then pour the mango puree on top.

3. Leave to set in the refrigerator for at least 30 minutes. Garnish with shredded coconut.

> The seeds for the pudding need to soak for at least 30 minutes, so ideally prepare this breakfast dish the night before. If pushed for time, just allow the chia seeds to soak for 10–15 minutes; the pudding will not be as firmly set.

QUINOA PUDDING

SERVES 2

½ cup (100 g) white **quinoa**
generous ¾ cup (200 ml) unsweetened rice milk
1 pinch vanilla powder or seeds
1 tsp (5 ml) agave syrup
7 oz (200 g) strawberries
1 tbsp (6 g) sliced almonds

NUTRITIONAL VALUE
per portion

kcal	kJ	Protein	Fat	Carbo-hydrate
240	1,020	8	6	39

1. Rinse the quinoa well under cold running water until it runs clear, then drain.

2. Heat the rice milk and vanilla in a pan with the agave syrup. Add the quinoa and simmer on low heat for about 10 minutes, stirring occasionally.

3. Rinse the strawberries briefly, remove the stems, and chop the flesh into small pieces. Set a few aside for garnish, then fold the rest into the cooked quinoa.

4. Divide the quinoa pudding between two glasses or bowls, and garnish with chopped strawberries and sliced almonds.

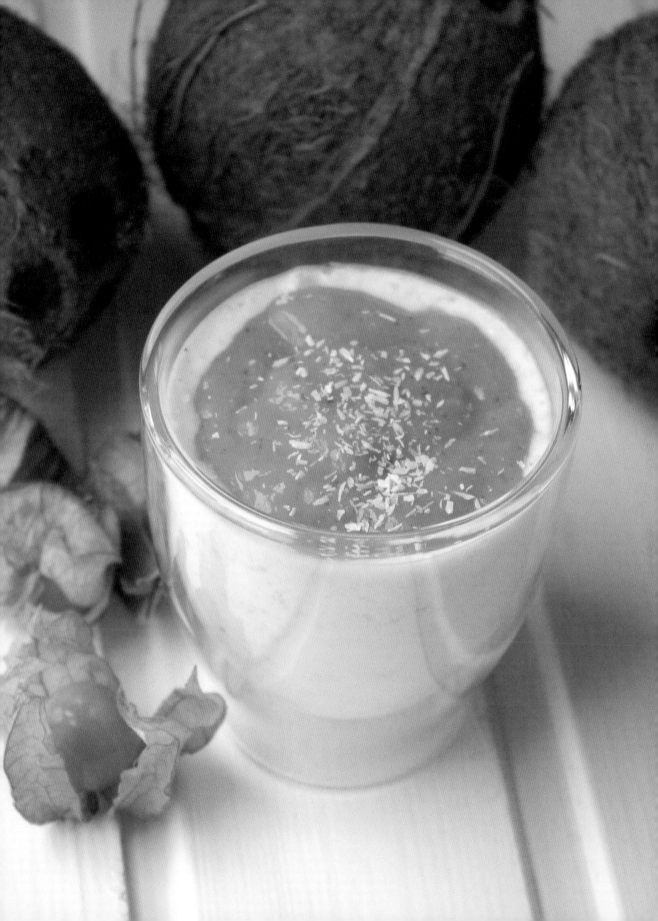

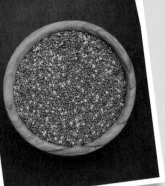

CHIA SEEDS

Small, but highly nutritious: Native to Mexico, chia seeds were a basic food source and energy provider in the Maya and Aztec diet thousands of years ago. These tiny black or white seeds, which are now widely regarded as a superfood, come from several varieties of sage (mainly *Salvia hispanica*). The high antioxidant content of these "antiaging seeds" protects our cells from free radicals, and this in turn can prevent many of the diseases associated with modern life. Their high levels of dietary fiber are also good for the digestion and have a detoxifying effect. When liquid is added to the seeds they swell up, turning them into "chia gel." Their mucilaginous polysaccharide coating gives a long-lasting feeling of being full and prevents snacking. Last but not least, chia seeds are high in omega-3 fatty acids. Eating them regularly can help lower the cholesterol level, blood pressure, and blood fats. Their high protein content gives an energy boost and promotes muscle development. They also contain minerals like calcium, potassium, iron, and magnesium—chia seeds are fantastic little bundles of energy! The clue is actually in the name itself: "chia" means "strength" in Nahuatl, the language of the Aztec people.

Ground Flaxseeds

Flaxseeds, also known as linseeds, are a homegrown alternative. They are equally good for improving the digestion, without all the air-mile baggage. However, chia seeds contain more antioxidants and omega-3 fatty acids. The polysaccharide layer of flaxseeds is found inside the hulls rather than on top of the seeds, so they should be crushed or freshly ground before eating them, or else the body will not be able to fully process the nutrients (see also flaxseed oil, p. 67).

USES

As chia seeds are flavor-neutral, they are used in a variety of ways for both sweet and savory dishes: in muesli, yogurt, porridge, overnight oats (p. 28), chia pudding (p. 14), or smoothies. They also work well as garnish for salads and in baking. Chia jam (p. 12) can be made very quickly, without added sugar or any cooking. The seeds are also used as a thickener in sauces and soups (pumpkin soup with chia, p. 82). To make **chia gel** as a thickening agent (e.g. for smoothies or desserts), grind the whole seeds in a blender, or with a mortar and pestle and mix with six times the amount of water or (soy) milk, then leave to soak for at least 30 minutes in the refrigerator. As an **egg substitute**, calculate 1 tablespoon of chia seeds plus 3 tablespoons of water for each egg.

GOJI BERRIES

In China, the main cultivation area for goji berries, this sweet-and-sour berry fruit has been a favorite ingredient in many dishes for thousands of years.

In traditional Chinese medicine (TCM), the "antiaging berry" is one of the most important remedies for health, performance, and vitality. Among the many conditions it has traditionally been used to treat are high blood pressure, eye disorders, exhaustion, tinnitus, dizziness, and a weakened immune system. Goji berries are regarded as a basic tonic for the organism as a whole, and they are reputed to improve liver function, the blood count, and skin complexion. In the West, there is debate about their properties and medical effectiveness, for which there is no scientific proof. Numerous studies into these "wonder berries" are currently under way in different countries. The "most nutritious fruit in the world" is said to contain 21 key minerals and trace elements, 19 amino acids, and large amounts of antioxidants and essential fatty acids. What is beyond dispute is that the berries have a high content of vitamins A (beta-carotene), C, and the B complex, as well as a whole host of antioxidants. As they have wide-ranging preventive benefits for our health, they now rank among the superfoods in our diet.

Goji berries are also easy to grow in our own backyards, though this large bush does need some space. Low maintenance and frost-hardy, this plant has been cultivated in Europe and North America for many years, mostly as an ornamental shrub or to reinforce the soil on freeways or embankments. The plant is known by a number of names including Chinese boxthorn, Chinese wolfberry, or barbary matrimony vine (*Lycium barbarum*) and the fruits sometimes as "wolfberries." It has attracted significant attention in the West only since the goji berry boom.

Warning: Medical authorities have warned of potentially dangerous interactions between goji berries and blood-thinning anticoagulant medications and an associated increased risk of hemorrhaging.

USES

As well as being used to make juice, goji berries find their way into muesli, nut mixtures, yogurt, and smoothies. These tangy fruits also taste great in baked goods, or as a topping for salads, desserts, or breakfast dishes (banana splits, p. 126; superfruit proats, p. 26). They also work well in game, poultry, and rice dishes, and are available commercially in the form of jams and fruit teas.

STRAWBERRY AND CHOCOLATE SMOOTHIE WITH MACA

MAKES approx. 2 cups (½ liter)
5½ oz (150 g) strawberries
1 banana
1 pinch vanilla powder or seeds
1 tsp (3 g) **maca powder**
generous ¾ cup (200 ml)
unsweetened almond milk
1 tbsp (8 g) **cocoa nibs**

NUTRITIONAL VALUE

per portion

kcal	kJ	Protein	Fat	Carbo-hydrate
100	410	2	2	17

1. Wash the strawberries under cold running water and drain. Remove the stems and cut the strawberries in half.

2. Peel and chop the banana. Whizz to a puree in a blender along with the strawberries, vanilla, maca, and almond milk.

3. Pour the smoothie into two large tumblers and garnish with the cocoa nibs.

When strawberries are out of season I prefer to use frozen ones. However, a powerful blender is essential when using frozen fruit. The smoothie can then be eaten with a spoon.

MUESLI SMOOTHIE

MAKES approx. 2 cups (½ liter)
1 small apple
1¾ oz (50 g) fresh berries, mixed if you like
2 tbsp (15 g) shelled **walnuts**
¼ cup (20 g) traditional rolled oats
1½ cups (350 ml) unsweetened oat milk
rolled oats or nuts for garnish

NUTRITIONAL VALUE

per portion

kcal	kJ	Protein	Fat	Carbo-hydrate
220	910	10	8	26

1. Wash and quarter the apple, remove the seeds, and chop the flesh. Rinse the berries briefly and drain. Coarsely chop the shelled walnuts.

2. Whizz all the ingredients in a blender until smooth. Divide the smoothie between two tumblers.

3. Garnish to taste with oat flakes or nuts and serve with a spoon.

The rolled oats and walnuts make the muesli smoothie especially filling and nutritious. As well as vitamins and carbohydrates, the walnuts also contain healthy fats. Out of the berry season, other types of fruit or frozen berries can be used. If you use less oat milk or more rolled oats, you can eat this breakfast dish with a spoon.

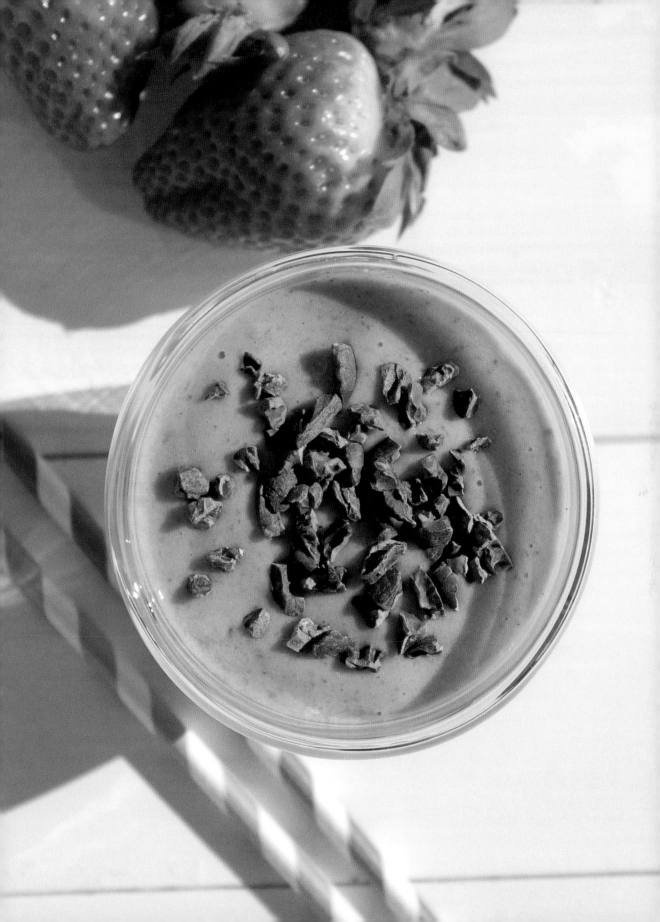

KALE SMOOTHIE

WITH PINEAPPLE

MAKES approx. 2 cups (½ liter)
1 handful **kale** (approx.
2½ oz/75 g)
½ banana
1 slice pineapple
(approx. 1¾ oz/50 g)

NUTRITIONAL VALUE

per portion

kcal	kJ	Protein	Fat	Carbo-hydrate
60	260	2	0	12

1. Remove the stems and tough veins from the kale, then wash, drain, and coarsely chop the leaves.

2. Peel and finely chop the banana and pineapple.

3. Whizz all the ingredients in a blender with 1¼ cups (300 ml) of water until smooth. Divide the smoothie between two tumblers.

> Spinach makes a good substitute for kale. Coconut water instead of plain water gives the smoothie a really delicate flavor.

WHITE SMOOTHIE

MAKES approx. 2 cups (½ liter)
1 ripe banana
1 tsp (3 g) **maca powder**
1 tbsp (8 g) hulled **hemp seeds**
1 tbsp (15 ml) **coconut oil**
1½ cups (350 ml) **coconut milk** or
coconut water (see text box)
shredded coconut for garnish

NUTRITIONAL VALUE

per portion

kcal	kJ	Protein	Fat	Carbo-hydrate
140	590	2	8	15

1. Peel and finely chop the banana. Whizz in a blender with the maca, hemp seeds, coconut oil, and coconut milk. Divide between two tumblers and garnish with the shredded coconut.

> A clean coconut milk should only contain coconut and water. To make your own, whizz freshly chopped coconut and coconut water in a blender. Shredded coconut can also be used: Simply cover it with two to four times the amount of boiling water in the mixer. Whizz until smooth, leave it to stand for about 15 minutes, then pass it through a fine sieve or muslin. If you use fresh coconut, you can leave the solids in the milk if you like. Homemade coconut milk will keep for about 2 days in a well-sealed container in the refrigerator.

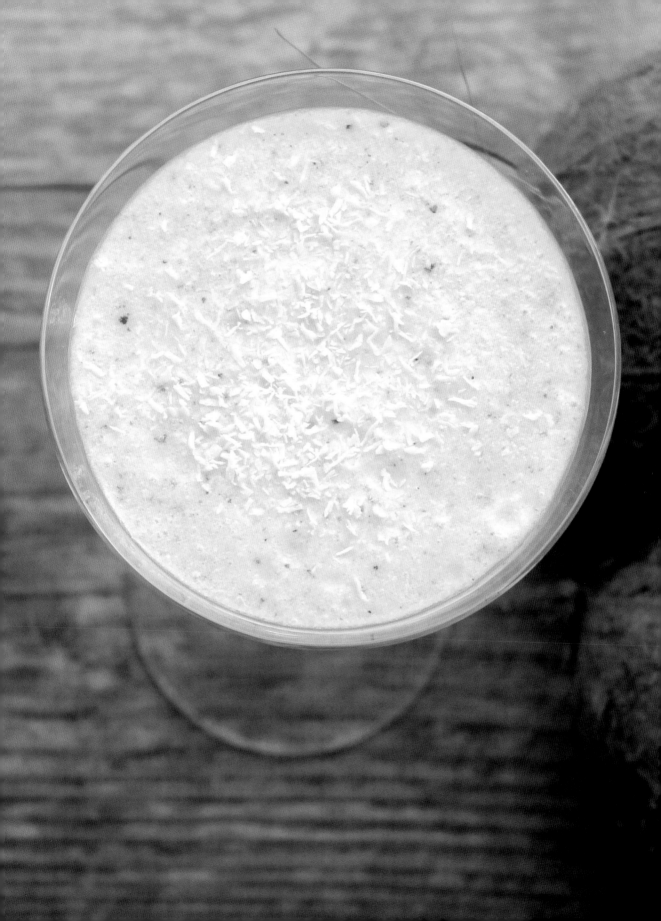

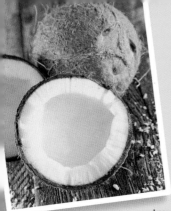

COCONUT

Coconut water is now well established as a trendy drink in the United States and is becoming increasingly popular in Europe as well. This liquid contained inside young, green coconuts (*Cocos nucifera*) is very rich in minerals, especially magnesium, potassium, phosphorus, selenium, calcium, and iron. It is naturally isotonic and is similar in composition to our blood plasma. As a low-calorie isotonic drink, coconut water provides the perfect fluid supply. It is also sold commercially mixed with other juices, extracts, or concentrates, but the quality of pure coconut water beats them all!

The same applies to **coconut milk**: Make sure that it contains only coconut and water. Coconut milk is the **fruit pulp** mixed with water, then pressed and filtered. It is a particularly nutritious energy source, contains plenty of fiber, and about one-third of it is made up of the fat, **coconut oil**. Despite a very high level of saturated fat, the oil is claimed by many to be very healthy. It contains approximately 45 percent lauric acid, which can raise the HDL level ("good cholesterol"). Coconut oil is easily digested and converted into energy by the body without resulting in weight gain. It also helps to protect against bacteria, viruses, fungal infection, and parasites, boosting the immune system. Its application in other areas is currently being debated, including the treatment of cardiovascular disease, diabetes, and fatigue, as well as for strengthening teeth, bones, skin, and hair. A balanced diet consists of coconut oil alternated with other oils containing unsaturated fatty acids. Organic virgin coconut oil should be used if possible in order to avoid harmful trans fats.

Coconut flour is also produced from coconut meat. It is very rich in fiber and protein, good for the digestion, low in calories, and tastes great (see below).

USES

Fresh coconut tastes great on its own as a snack, in fruit salads, yogurt, and desserts. Coconut milk is often used in curries, soups, and sauces, but is also great in desserts (chia pudding with coconut milk and mango, p. 14). Coconut milk and coconut water work well in smoothies and other drinks (coconut and raspberry smoothie, p. 24; white smoothie, p. 20). Coconut oil is very heat-stable (to 390 °F/200 °C), making it an ideal fat for baking, roasting, and deep-frying. Coconut flour acts as a binding agent in soups and sauces. As it is gluten-free, you can replace up to a third of other grain flours with it in many baking recipes. As coconut flour absorbs a lot of liquid, you will need to use far more than usual. The flour has a very delicate, sweet flavor.

ARONIA BERRIES
Black Chokeberries

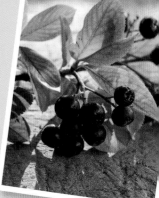

Aronia berries (*Aronia melanocarpa*), also known as black chokeberries, were relatively unknown outside North America until this century. They have become a trendy fruit, with some justification. They contain by far the highest levels of antioxidants (anthocyanins and flavonoids) of any fruit, and consequently the highest ORAC value (see p. 6). This means that the aronia berry is especially valuable for protecting our cells from free radicals. According to current research and long-term studies, the regular consumption of aronia berries can protect our bodies and immune systems from many diseases, including cardiovascular disease, diabetes, cancer, and stomach and liver conditions. These berries are also packed full of vital substances: vitamins C, E, K, and the B complex; a remarkably high amount of folic acid, iron, and iodine; and magnesium, calcium, and potassium. Aronia berries are native to North America, where they formed an important part of the Native American diet. They are now widely cultivated in many countries, especially Eastern Europe. The plants are increasingly found in our own gardens, as the aronia bush is a very hardy, frost-resistant, and low-maintenance plant. Attractive, space-saving standard varieties are now available as well.

Make sure that fresh berries are fully ripe, when the flesh is a deep red color. Only then do the berries contain the maximum level of healthy substances and their flavor is at its best. Fresh berries are in season in the fall. As the berries keep for up to two weeks, they are sometimes sold by mail order, and they freeze well for storage. Aronia berries are usually available in frozen or powdered form, or as a juice.

Aronia seeds contain small amounts of prussic acid, a toxic compound that is also found in apple seeds and apricot pits. The toxin is rendered harmless by processing (when dried, heated, or made into juice). You should, however, avoid eating very large quantities of the fresh berries raw.

USES

Aronia berries have a sharp, tangy flavor, with a hint of bitter almond. The fresh fruit is made into juice, syrup, jam, or fruit sauce. In dried form, they are used for smoothies, fruit bars, or raw fruit pralines. They can be added straight to muesli, yogurt, overnight oats (p. 28), or proats (p. 26). I like to use them as a topping. To make one cup of **aronia tea**, pour boiling water over 1 tablespoon of dried aronia berries and leave them to infuse for 8 to 10 minutes.

COCONUT AND RASPBERRY SMOOTHIE

MAKES approx. 2 cups (½ liter)
5½ oz (150 g) raspberries
1¼ cups (300 ml) **coconut milk**
1 tsp (5 ml) **coconut oil**
1 tsp (3 g) **maca powder**
¼ cup (20 g) rolled oat flakes
1 pinch vanilla powder or seeds
shredded coconut for garnish

1. Rinse the raspberries briefly and drain them. Whizz the coconut milk, coconut oil, maca, oats, vanilla, and raspberries in a blender until smooth.

2. Divide the smoothie between two tumblers and garnish with the shredded coconut.

NUTRITIONAL VALUE
per portion

kcal	kJ	Protein	Fat	Carbo-hydrate
140	570	3	8	12

ACAI AND BLUEBERRY SMOOTHIE

SERVES 2
½ banana
1¼ cups (300 ml) unsweetened
plant-based milk (e.g. almond milk)
7 oz (200 g) fresh **blueberries**
1 tsp (3 g) **acai powder**
goji berries and pollen
granules for garnish

1. Peel and finely chop the banana. Whizz together with the milk, washed blueberries, and acai powder in a blender until smooth.

2. Divide the smoothie between two tumblers and garnish with the goji berries and pollen granules.

> Blackberries also work well instead of blueberries: They make the smoothie even sweeter.

NUTRITIONAL VALUE
per portion

kcal	kJ	Protein	Fat	Carbo-hydrate
90	380	2	2	14

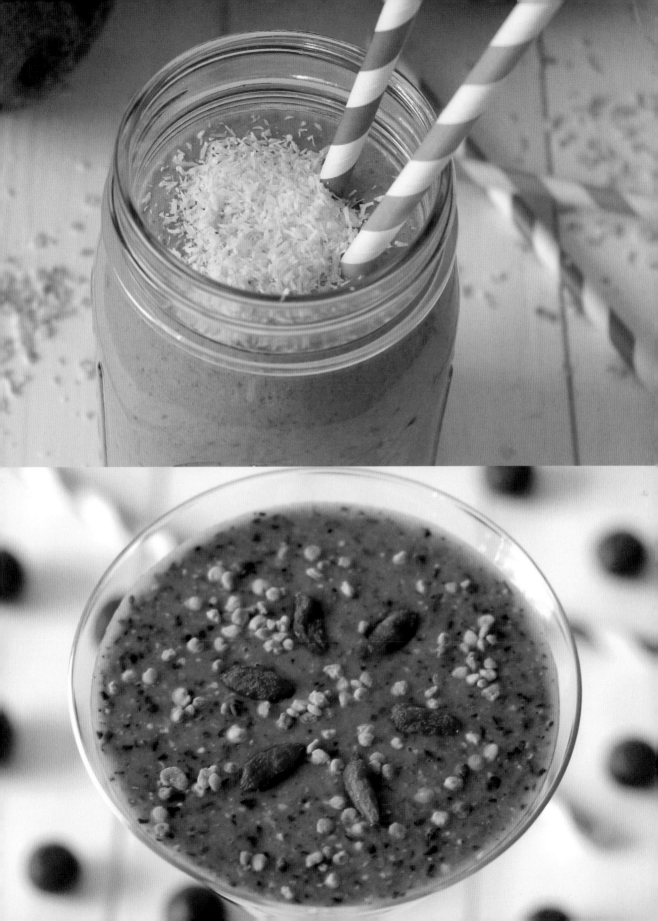

RED SUPERFRUIT PROATS

SERVES 2

generous ¾ cup (80 g)
rolled oat flakes
7 oz (200 g) strawberries
9 tbsp (150 g) Greek,
natural, or soy yogurt
1 tbsp (8 g) unsweetened
cranberries
1 tbsp (8 g) dried **goji berries**
1 tbsp (8 g) dried unsweetened
barberries (see text box)

NUTRITIONAL VALUE
per portion

kcal	kJ	Protein	Fat	Carbo-hydrate
290	1,200	9	11	38

1. Bring a generous ¾ cup (200 ml) of water to a boil in a small pan. Add the oat flakes and simmer for 5 minutes, stirring occasionally.

2. Wash the strawberries under cold running water and remove the stems. Whizz 4 oz (120 g) of the strawberries and the yogurt in a blender until smooth. Slice the rest of the strawberries and set them to one side.

3. Combine the strawberry yogurt with the oat flakes and divide the mixture between two small bowls.

4. Serve with the remaining strawberries, and the cranberries, goji berries, and barberries.

Although **barberries** are grown throughout Europe and North America, they are mainly known today because of their use in Persian and Indian cuisine. These sour berries are very rich in vitamin C, and their juice was formerly used as a substitute for lemon juice. Barberries are believed to be an effective remedy against poisoning in Ayurvedic medicine. The dried fruit can be used just like raisins and are ideal for baking. They are often available on supermarket shelves in the summer months.

"**Proats**" (a combination of "protein" and "oats") are tasty as well as easy to prepare, healthy, and filling. Cow's or plant-based milk is brought to a boil and mixed with Greek yogurt, which is particularly high in protein. Alternatively, you can of course use ordinary natural yogurt or a soy-based one instead.

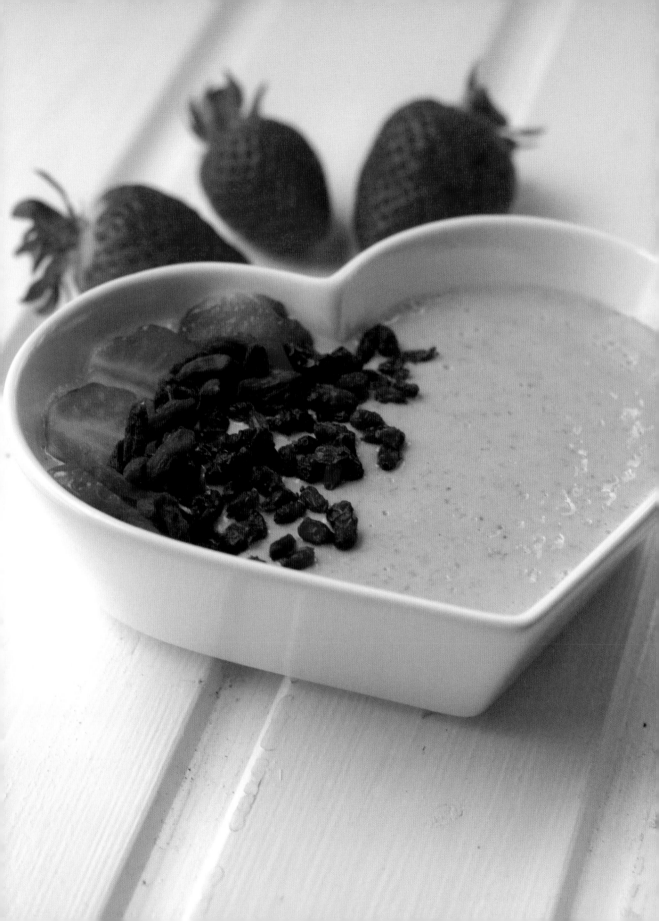

OVERNIGHT OATS

CHOCOLATE AND RASPBERRY

SERVES 2

1 cup (240 ml)
unsweetened oat milk
2 tsp (4 g) raw **cocoa powder**
generous ¾ cup (80 g)
rolled oat flakes
4½ oz (125 g) raspberries
generous ⅔ cup (175 g)
Greek or soy yogurt
2 tbsp (16 g) **cocoa nibs**

NUTRITIONAL VALUE

per portion

kcal	kJ	Protein	Fat	Carbo-hydrate
330	1,390	15	14	34

1. The previous evening, combine the oat milk, cocoa powder, and oat flakes in a bowl. Pick over the raspberries; rinse briefly and drain. In another bowl, mash together the raspberries and yogurt with a fork.

2. Divide the oat and cocoa mixture between two glasses or bowls, then pour the raspberry yogurt on top.

3. Cover the oats and chill overnight in the refrigerator. Before serving, garnish with the cocoa nibs.

> To make quick and healthy **overnight oats**, soak 1 part oat flakes to 3 parts liquid in the refrigerator overnight.

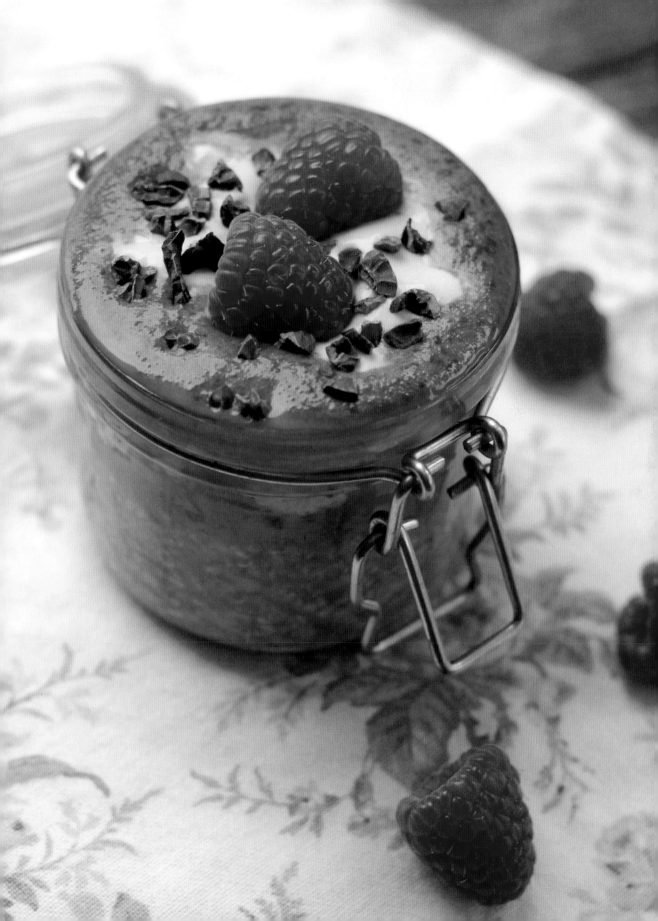

MATCHA AND BANANA MILK SHAKE

MAKES approx. 2 cups (½ liter)
1 ripe banana
1½ cups (350 ml)
unsweetened almond milk
1 tsp (3 g) **matcha powder**
2 tbsp (10 g) rolled oat flakes

NUTRITIONAL VALUE
per portion

kcal	kJ	Protein	Fat	Carbo-hydrate
120	520	3	3	21

1. Peel and finely chop the banana. Whizz in a blender with the almond milk, matcha powder, and oat flakes until smooth.

2. Pour the milk shake into two tumblers. Sprinkle with a little matcha powder to taste.

> If you prefer your shake a little sweeter, add some agave syrup. Vanilla or finely grated ginger work well too, and in summer you can blend in some ice cubes.

MATCHA PROATS

WITH BANANA FOAM

SERVES 2
generous ¾ cup (80 g) rolled oat flakes
10 tbsp (150 g) Greek,
natural, or soy yogurt
1 tsp (3 g) **matcha powder**
1 banana
7 tbsp (100 ml) unsweetened
almond milk
1 pinch vanilla powder or seeds
1 tbsp (8 g) dried unsweetened
barberries (see p. 26)

NUTRITIONAL VALUE
per portion

kcal	kJ	Protein	Fat	Carbo-hydrate
290	1,220	9	11	39

1. Bring generous ¾ cup (200 ml) of water to a boil in a small pan. Add the oat flakes and simmer for 5 minutes, stirring occasionally.

2. Combine the yogurt and matcha in a small mixing bowl. Fold in the oat flakes and divide between 2 small serving bowls.

3. Peel and chop the banana. Whizz in a blender with the almond milk and vanilla, then pour it over the matcha proats. Garnish with barberries.

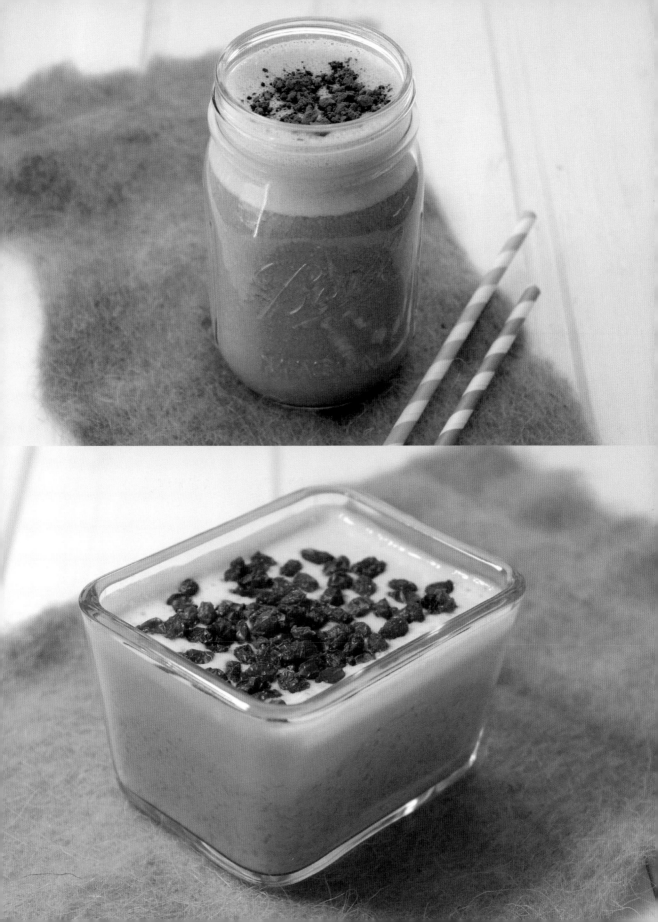

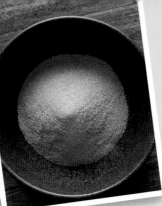

MATCHA

Matcha is a very finely ground green tea that is complicated to produce. The plants grow slowly in shaded plantations so they form lots of chlorophyll. The leaves are harvested by hand, steamed, dried, and carefully picked over—sometimes even the leaf veins and stems are removed. Finally, they are ground to a fine powder in a granite mill—all of which explains the high price tag. When buying matcha from a store, look for organic matcha from Japan. Other types have often been produced with less care and refinement, or even cut with "ordinary" green tea. There is no comparison when it comes to taste and effects. Matcha is supposed to be a vibrant green color—a pale or yellowish green is by contrast a sure sign of poor quality.

Matcha is currently trending as a stimulant. It contains more caffeine than coffee and has the same invigorating effect, but this is balanced out by its amino acids content. This refined green tea is comparatively easier to digest and has a more calming effect than coffee. Matcha contains vitamins A, C, and E, minerals and dietary fiber; it is also rich in antioxidants, which explains its high ORAC value. It also contains the active agent epigallocatechin gallate (EGCG), an anti-inflammatory that can have a positive effect on diseases of the immune system and cancer, according to research by the University of Colorado. This "in" drink is also believed to help with weight loss and muscle development, and to delay the aging process in skin. Unlike standard green tea, matcha is not imbibed as an infusion. The whole leaf is consumed: Pour ⅓ cup (80 ml) of warm water (175 °F/80 °C) over a ½ teaspoon (1.5 g) of matcha and mix until frothy using either a bamboo whisk or an electric milk frother.

USES

Matcha can be used to make tea or in cooking and baking. The powder is light-sensitive and should be stored in a cool, dark place. Its grassy note goes well with both sweet and savory dishes. The strong green color is popular as a natural food coloring. So a "cooking matcha" is available for this purpose that is of a lower grade and cheaper. Matcha makes a very good stimulant at breakfast time in particular (matcha proats with banana foam, p. 30). It also adds an extra dimension to smoothies and shakes (matcha and banana milk shake, p. 30). A classic dish in Japanese restaurants is matcha ice cream. Matcha on the rocks (a nonalcoholic cocktail) and **matcha latte** are becoming extremely popular in the West: To make the latte, simply add ⅓ cup (80 ml) of hot water (175 °F/80 °C) to ½ teaspoon (1.5 g) of matcha powder in a tumbler, and mix it until frothy with a whisk or milk frother. Add a generous ¾ cup (200 ml) of frothed (plant-based) milk.

BLUEBERRIES

These little berries are real powerhouses for our immune system: There are high levels of anthocyanins in their purple-blue plant pigment. Their extremely high antioxidant content makes blueberries (*Vaccinium myrtillus* and *Vaccinium corymbosum*) one of today's superfoods. They protect the body and our cells against free radicals and many diseases, and are said to be especially effective against cardio-vascular disease and high blood pressure. A study by Swedish scientists at the University of Lund has confirmed that blueberries can prevent and alleviate inflammation of the bowel, a traditional remedy in folk medicine. And even a handful of the berries each day can measurably help maintain the memory and learning abilities into old age, according to a study by Boston University. If blueberries are eaten regularly, their high content of beta-carotene is believed to result in improved vision function in darkness. They also contain lots of vitamins C, E, some of the B complex, and minerals like tannic acid. Dried blueberries are a traditional remedy for diarrhea, while the fresh berries are good for the digestion. Gargling with the warm juice of the plant is said to be a scientifically proven treatment for inflammation in the mouth and throat areas.

The healthiest way to eat blueberries is in their natural, unprocessed form. Wild blueberries, with their blue, staining flesh, contain far higher amounts of anthocyanins than the pale flesh of cultivated garden plants. Blueberries grow wild in the high reaches of low mountain ranges and on heaths. They can also be grown in your garden, though you will have to create a soil area with ericaceous compost to be successful. The peak blueberry season in North America is June and July.

USES

The sweet, intense aroma of the fresh berries is enjoyed best in its natural form in (soy) yogurt or quark, creams, and smoothies (acai and blueberry smoothie, p. 24). Blueberries are a popular ingredient in baking and are used for cakes, tarts, and muffins. They can be made into juice, syrup, bowls, jam, or sauce. The berries also work well in savory dishes like salad, for instance.

ACAI BOWL

WITH ORANGE

MAKES approx. 2 cups (½ liter)
scant 1¼ cups (300 g)
yogurt, preferably soy
1 tsp (3 g) **acai powder**
2 tbsp (15 g) puffed **quinoa**
1 orange
1 tsp (8 g) **chia seeds**
1 tsp (8 g) sesame seeds
dried **mulberries** for garnish

NUTRITIONAL VALUE

per portion

kcal	kJ	Protein	Fat	Carbo-hydrate
110	470	7	3	12

1. Combine the yogurt and acai powder in a bowl, and fold in the puffed quinoa. Cut the orange in half horizontally, and squeeze the juice from one half. Stir the orange juice into the yogurt mixture.

2. Peel the other orange half. Cut the flesh into small pieces.

3. Divide the yogurt mixture between two bowls and garnish with chopped orange, chia seeds, sesame seeds, and mulberries.

An acai bowl is a popular breakfast across the United States, especially in Hawaii and California for instance. "Bowls" also taste great with nut or coconut milk instead of yogurt, and the acai berries give the dish its lovely pink to purple color.

Puffed quinoa can be bought ready-made in stores, but it can be made at home quickly as well. Simply heat a large pot until very hot and add 1 tablespoon of quinoa. Cover the pot with a lid. As soon as the grains begin to pop, remove the pot from the stove and shake it gently back and forward.

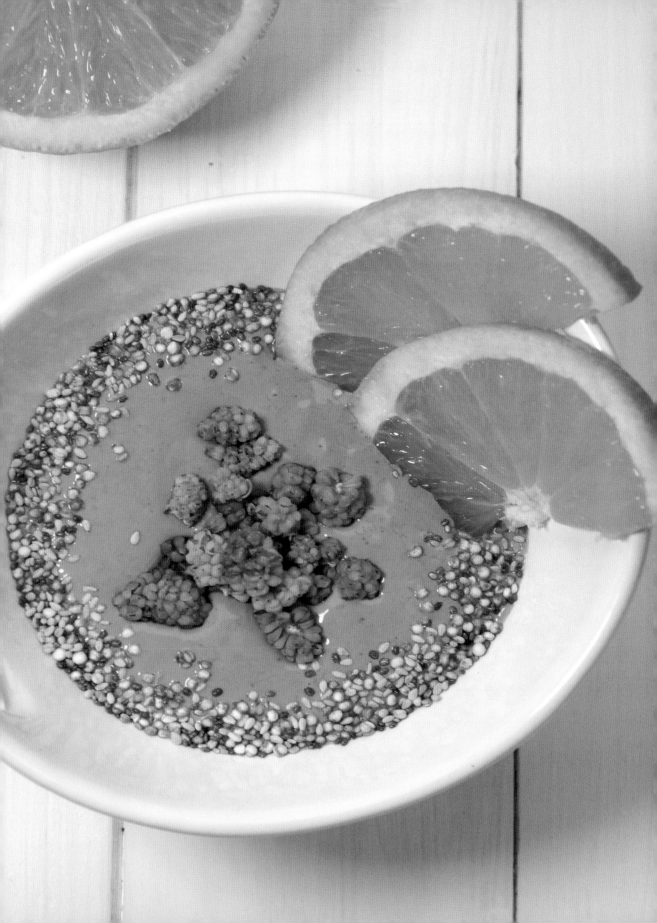

ACAI BERRIES

Acai berries (pronounced "ah-sigh-ee") are a dark blue to deep purple-black color. They are native to the Amazon rainforest, where they grow on acai palms (*Euterpe oleracea*) as high as 66 ft (20 m). Freshly picked, they are eaten raw as berries or squeezed to make juice. In some cultivation areas they form a staple part of the diet, eaten in various forms almost every day. The only edible part is the thin skin, not the large pit. There is very little fruit pulp in the acai berry. Unfortunately, the fresh berries spoil quickly, so they are dried and pulverized on site for export. The drying process is said to preserve 95 percent of the nutrients. Acai berries are available in tablet, powder, or capsule form. Personally, I use the powdered form or frozen acai fruit purees, which undergo the least processing and are therefore ideally suited to the "clean eating" concept. Naturally, it would be better to eat the berries fresh and unprocessed, but this is impossible outside the cultivation areas.

Acai berries are reputed to stimulate the fat-burning process and hence to promote weight loss. So far there has been no serious research to support this claim. It is unlikely that acai berries will suddenly get rid of the stubborn fat stores we have been accumulating over the years. You should avoid acai diet products altogether as they have no place in a clean eating approach. The same applies to energy drinks and convenience foods such as ice cream, sparkling wine, sorbet, or chocolate made with acai berries.

Acai berries have a high anthocyanin content, which gives them their purple color and acts as an antioxidant in our bodies. These free radical scavengers protect our cells, prevent illnesses, and can slow down the aging process. However, we should be skeptical about claims that acai berries are the "wrinkle killers" that the commercial industry would have us believe. The fact is nonetheless that acai berries are very healthy and give us plenty of energy. In addition to the high levels of antioxidants, they contain vitamins A and C, the B complex, magnesium, potassium, calcium, and iron.

USES

In powder form, acai berries go well in yogurt, muesli, and smoothies, for example in my acai and blueberry smoothie (p. 24) or in an acai bowl (p. 34). The powder can also be used to make baked goods and ice cream. Acai berries work well in hearty savory dishes (beet soup with acai, p. 58). *Au naturel*, the dried berry has a tangy, slightly earthy flavor, so it takes a bit for our Western palates to get used to it. Prepared properly, it adds an exotic dimension to food.

MULBERRIES

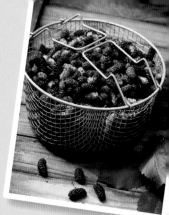

The ideal superfood if you have a sweet tooth! Mulberries (*Morus*) are very sweet, and not well known, for the moment at least. And yet this strange-looking berry bush has been cultivated in Europe since the 9th century. Today they can be seen mainly in parks and well-established gardens. The fact that they are not more widely grown is no doubt due to the poor shelf life of these berries, which are similar to blackberries. Juicy and easily bruised, they must be processed as soon as they have been harvested. For this reason, mulberries are usually available as dried fruit, pulp, or juice, and are black, white, or red in color. As a rule of thumb, when it comes to the red and black varieties, the darker the berries, the more intense is their sweet, fruity flavor.

What do these berries contain? As well as vitamin C and the B complex, they have iron, zinc, calcium, potassium, and magnesium. They also contain the latest nutritional sensation, the antioxidant resveratrol, which has been found in red grapes and red wine. There is scientific debate about their effectiveness against arteriosclerosis, cardiovascular disease, Alzheimer's, Parkinson's, diabetes, and arthritis. According to different studies, mulberries are said to have many health benefits in old age; to boost the fat-burning process; to lower blood pressure and blood sugar levels; and to improve muscle function. They are even believed to have cancer-inhibiting effects, as well as antibacterial and anti-inflammatory properties. Their application for coughs and throat inflammation is well known in traditional medicine. The leaves of the mulberry plant are also the subject of medical research and are available in tablet or extract form.

USES

If you have the rare chance to enjoy fresh mulberries, grab the opportunity to indulge in these aromatic, sweet berries with both hands. During harvest time (from August), it is wise to wear old clothes and gloves, as the berries cause bad staining. To prolong their shelf life, they can be easily boiled down into jam or syrup and used as a sweetener for desserts and smoothies. Dried mulberries usually have a crunchy, rather sticky consistency and taste really great in breakfast dishes, for example as a topping for muesli, yogurt, or overnight oats (see p. 28). They also work well in cake or muffin mixtures, and in fruit salads. I have also used them in my acai bowl (p. 34).

BERRY SMOOTHIE BOWL

SERVES 2

5½ oz (150 g) raspberries
1¾ oz (50 g) blackberries
generous ¾ cup (200 ml) soy milk
generous ¾ cup (80 g)
rolled oat flakes
2 tbsp (16 g) pumpkin seeds
2 tbsp (16 g) **chia seeds**
2 tbsp (16 g) sunflower seeds
2 tbsp (16) **goji berries**

NUTRITIONAL VALUE

per portion

kcal	kJ	Protein	Fat	Carbo-hydrate
270	1,130	14	9	33

1. Rinse the raspberries and blackberries briefly and drain them well. Reserve a handful of raspberries.

2. Whizz the remaining raspberries with the soy milk and oat flakes until smooth, and divide the mixture between two small bowls.

3. Garnish with pumpkin seeds, chia seeds, blackberries, sunflower seeds, and goji berries.

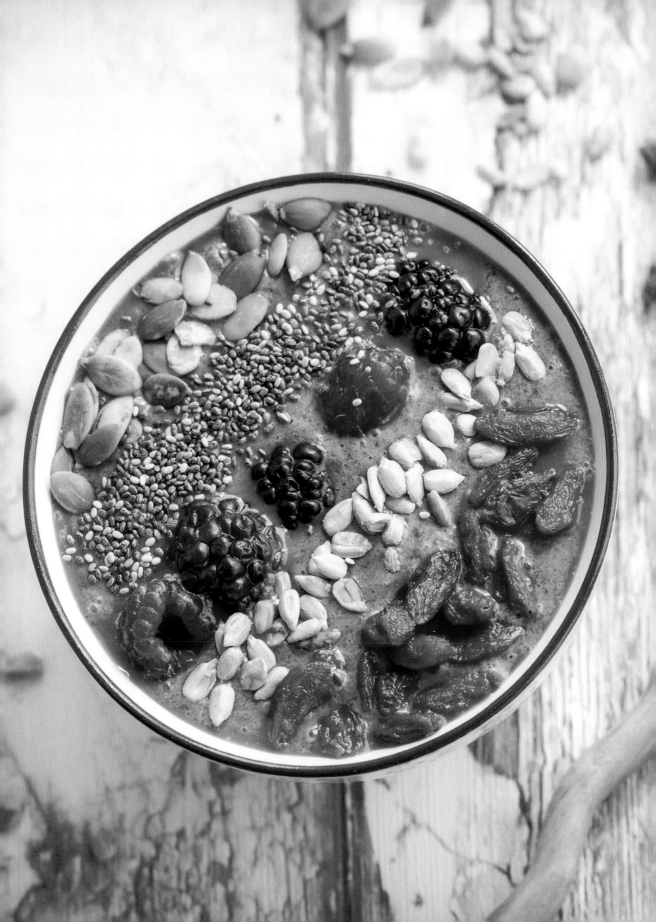

KHORASAN AND WALNUT ROLLS

MAKES 8

⅓ oz (10 g) fresh yeast
1 tsp (5 ml) agave syrup
2⅔ cups (400 g) khorasan
wheat flour
1 tbsp (15 ml) olive oil
salt
7 tbsp (50 g) shelled **walnuts**

NUTRITIONAL VALUE

per roll (when making 8)

kcal	kJ	Protein	Fat	Carbo-hydrate
214	897	7	7	31

1. The previous evening, crumble the yeast with your hands and dissolve it in the agave syrup with 3½ tablespoons (50 ml) of lukewarm water. Let it prove for 10 minutes.

2. Sieve the khorasan flour and add the yeast mixture, olive oil, salt, and a generous ¾ cup (200 ml) of lukewarm water. Knead it into a smooth dough, first with a food processor or the dough attachment of a hand mixer, and then with your hands. Coarsely chop the walnuts and work them into the dough.

3. Cover the dough with a tea towel and chill it overnight in the refrigerator. The next morning, divide the dough into eight pieces and shape them into rounds. Arrange them on a baking pan lined with wax paper and put them on the middle shelf of a cold oven.

4. Switch the oven on at 355 °F (180 °C) and bake the rolls for 8 minutes. Then finish baking the rolls for another 20 minutes at a slightly higher temperature.

AVOCADO SANDWICH TOPPING

SERVES 2

1 ripe **avocado**
juice of ½ **lemon**
1 tsp (5 ml) **flaxseed oil**
¼ tsp (0.5 g) chili powder or paprika
salt; freshly ground black pepper
some chili threads

NUTRITIONAL VALUE

per portion

kcal	kJ	Protein	Fat	Carbo-hydrate
170	730	2	17	5

1. Slice the avocado in half lengthways, twist the halves in opposite directions, and remove the pit. Scoop out the flesh with a spoon.

2. Whizz the avocado, lemon juice, flaxseed oil, chili powder, salt, and pepper in a blender until smooth.

3. Divide the topping between two slices of bread or two rolls, and garnish with chili threads.

> Very finely sliced chili threads make a decorative garnish and have quite a mild, fresh flavor.

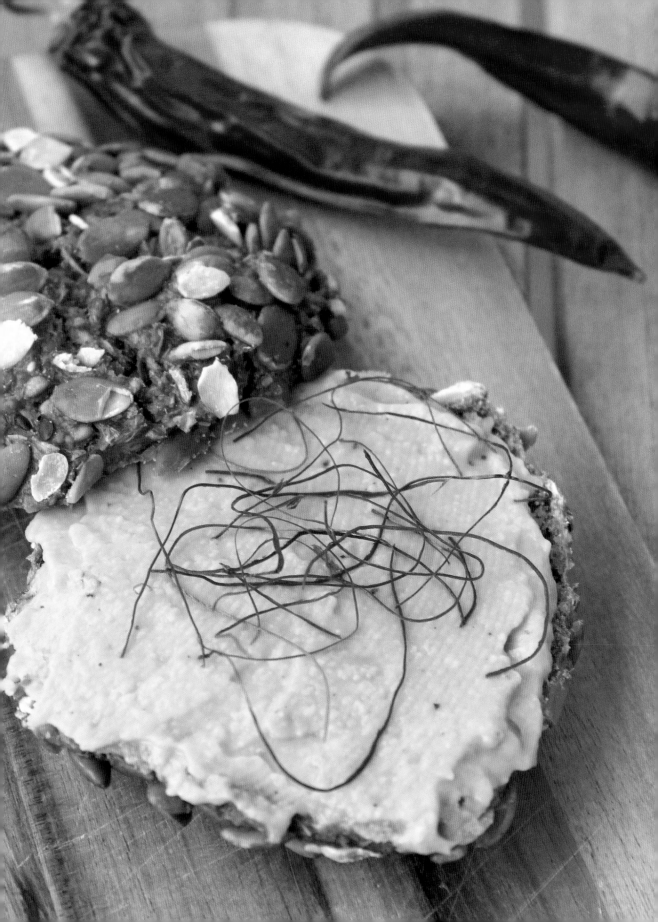

PUMPKIN BREAD

WITH HEMP SEEDS

FOR 1 baking pan
(approx. 6 × 10 in / 16 × 27 cm)
¾ lb (350 g) **hokkaido pumpkin**
2 tbsp (16 g) **hemp seeds,** hulled
generous 2 cups
(320 g) whole spelt flour
1½ tbsp (25 g) butter
or margarine
salt
1 tsp (5 ml) agave syrup
⅓ oz (10 g) fresh yeast

NUTRITIONAL VALUE per loaf

kcal	kJ	Protein	Fat	Carbo-hydrate
1,500	6,280	52	43	224

1. Wash the pumpkin, cut it in half with a sharp knife, and scoop the seeds out with a spoon. Weigh out the given amount and dice it, keeping the skin on.

2. Put it in a pan, cover with water, and bring to a boil. Cover with a lid and simmer gently for about 10 minutes until the pumpkin is soft. Drain off the water, whizz the pumpkin to a puree, and leave it to cool.

3. Dry-roast the hemp seeds briefly in a pan, stirring all the time. In a bowl, rub together the flour, butter, and salt.

4. Mix the agave syrup with the yeast and 3½ tablespoons (50 ml) of lukewarm water, then add it to the flour mixture. Add the pumpkin puree and hemp seeds, and knead it all into dough with your hands. Cover and leave to prove for 15 minutes.

5. Line a baking pan with wax paper. Transfer the dough to the pan, cover, and let it prove for another 30 minutes. Pre-heat the oven to 375 °F (190 °C).

6. Brush the bread with some water and bake in the pre-heated oven for 25–30 minutes (do a skewer test, see text box)

> To do a skewer test, stick a thin wooden skewer into the dough. If it comes out clean, the dough or cake is cooked.

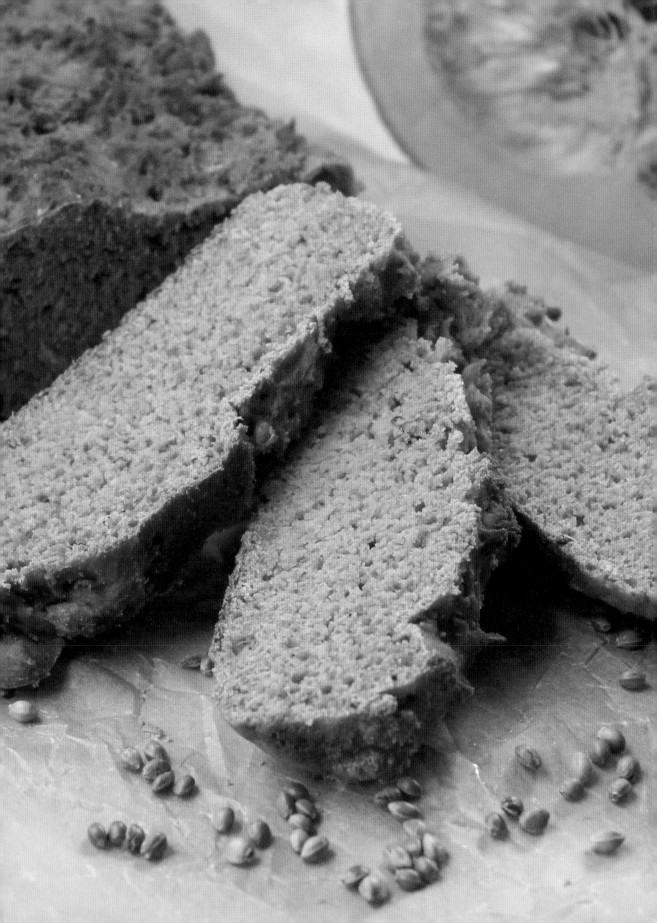

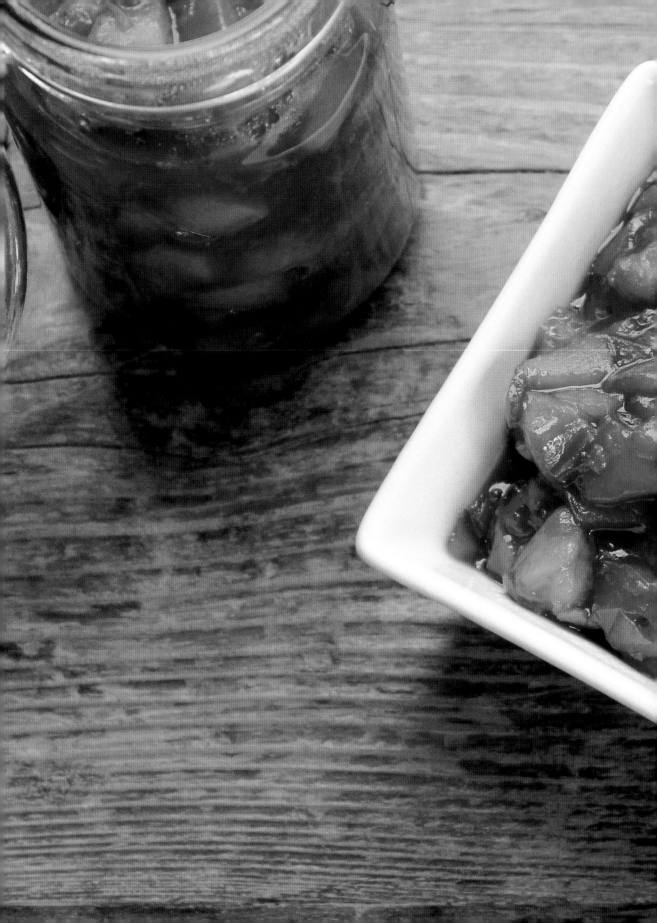

APPETIZERS

STUFFED DATES

WRAPPED IN ZUCCHINI

SERVES 2

6 fresh **dates**
1 small zucchini
2 tbsp (30 ml) olive oil
½ tsp (3 g) salt
2 tbsp (16 g) dried
unsweetened **cranberries**
2 tbsp (15 g) pine nuts

NUTRITIONAL VALUE

per portion

kcal	kJ	Protein	Fat	Carbo-hydrate
350	1,470	6	16	46

1. Slice into the dates lengthways and remove the pits.

2. Wash and trim the zucchini; cut it into six very thin slices with a sharp knife or mandoline.

3. Combine the oil and salt; soak the zucchini slices in it for about 10 minutes.

4. Coarsely chop the cranberries and pine nuts, then dry-roast them in a pan, stirring all the time. Using a teaspoon, fill the dates with this mixture. Close the dates and roll each one in a zucchini slice. Hold it in place with a cocktail stick.

5. Brown the little rolls all over in a pan, without adding any more oil, until golden, and serve.

You can also use eggplant instead of the zucchini.

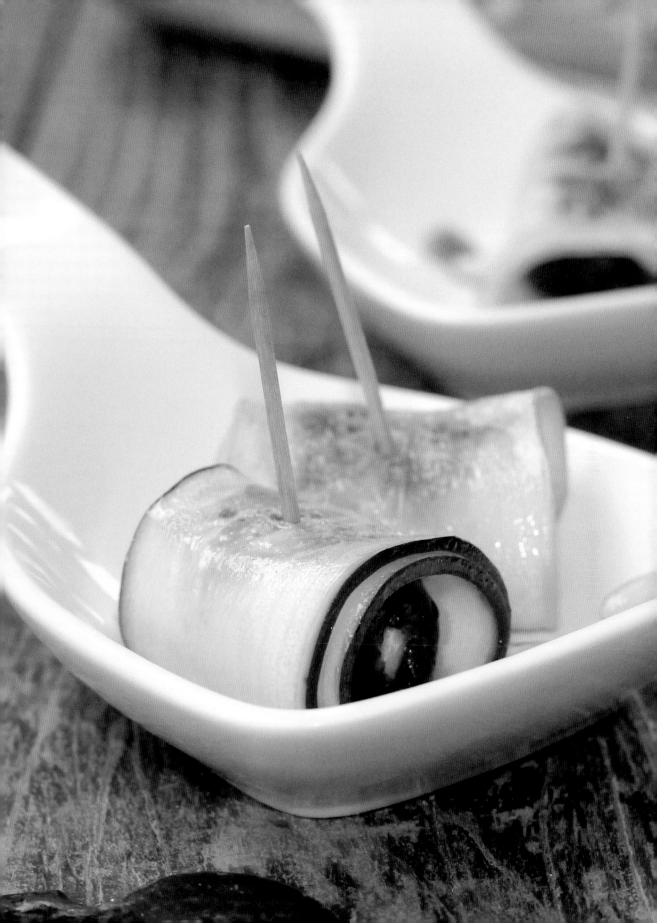

POMEGRANATE AND CUCUMBER BITES

SERVES 2

½ cucumber
⅓ cup (80 g) cream cheese
1 tsp (5 ml) honey
½ **pomegranate**
1 tsp (5 g) pollen granules
(see text box)

NUTRITIONAL VALUE

per portion

kcal	kJ	Protein	Fat	Carbo-hydrate
190	810	5	13	13

1. Wash the cucumber, and cut it into ten slices (approx. ½ in / 1 cm thick). Combine the cream cheese and honey, and spread it on top of the cucumber slices.

2. Remove the seeds from the pomegranate (see p.50) and arrange them on top of the cream cheese. Garnish with the pollen granules.

> You can also use goji berries instead of the pollen granules.

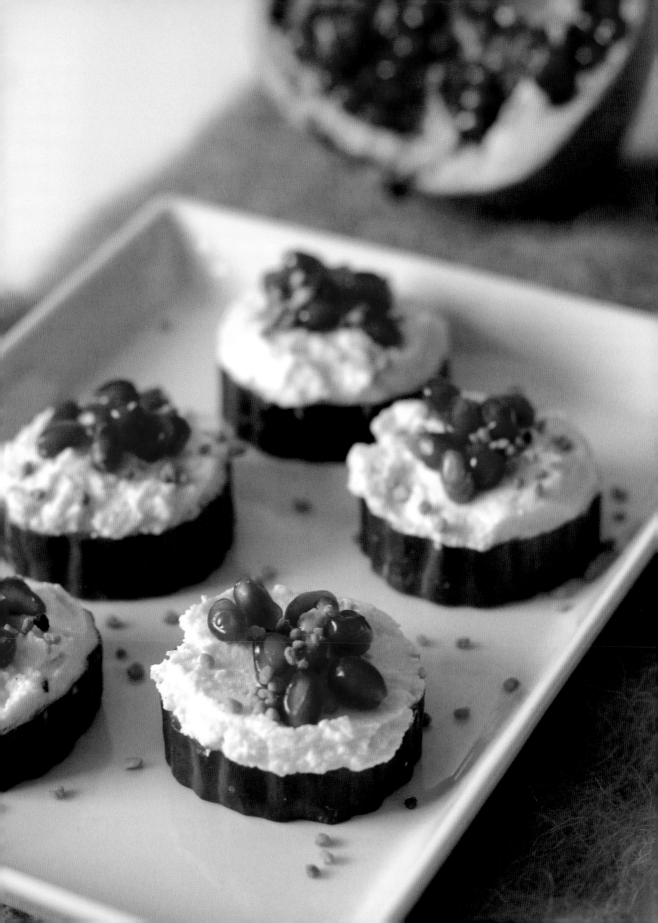

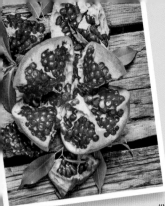

POMEGRANATE

An old Turkish riddle poses the question: "What is one on the outside and a thousand and one inside?" The answer is one of the oldest cultivated plants known to humankind—the pomegranate. As a symbol of life, fertility, beauty, and love, the fruit has been assigned special significance since biblical times. The pomegranate tree (*Punica granatum*) is still widely grown today, especially in West to Central Asia, the Near East, the Mediterranean, and southern United States. The beautiful red-orange blossoms catch our eye immediately, then we spot the bright-red, round fruits with their little "crown." They contain the red seeds (up to 400, in fact, in each fruit) that end up as the showstoppers on our plates.

Pomegranate seeds contain lots of potassium, calcium, iron, and B vitamins, and are rich in antioxidant flavonoids and anthocyanins. These provide the red color in the seeds and peel, and their pigment is so strong that it was formerly used for dying Indian wool and Oriental carpets. Yellow pomegranates are also available, most of which come from Spain.

According to recent research, pomegranates can boost the body's resistance, lower blood pressure, and prevent cardiovascular disease. Their cancer-inhibiting properties have been the subject of many studies, and their inclusion in the diet has been recommended by some in cases of breast and prostate cancer. There is debate about their medical effectiveness, for which there is currently no scientific proof.

USES

The pomegranate—with its sweet-and-sour red "fruit pearls"—is in season from September to February in the West. To **open the fruit**, cut off the stem end (crown) and carve a cross into the fruit with a knife. Then break it up under water in a bowl using your hands. This prevents the juice from squirting out, as it leaves stubborn stains. The seeds sink to the bottom of the bowl, while the peel and membranes float to the top for skimming off. Only the seeds are used, everything else is discarded. To make **pomegranate juice**, cut the fruit in half with a knife and squeeze the juice out of each half using a lemon juicer: one pomegranate produces about 7 tablespoons (100 ml) of juice. When you buy pomegranate juice commercially, look for brands that are sugar-free, preferably organic, and not from concentrate. Pomegranate seeds are used in desserts and fruit salads (superfruit salad, p. 138) as well as in savory dishes (quinoa tabbouleh, p. 68; pomegranate and cucumber bites, p. 48). They also give an extra dimension to fruit spreads, salads, and smoothies.

AVOCADO

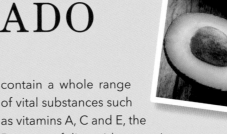

In botanical terms, the avocado (*Persea americana*) is actually a berry that grows on a tree, not a vegetable. It was regarded as a luxury in the West until the 1980s, but now you will find it on every supermarket shelf.

This power-packed fruit contains up to 30 percent fat, more than any other fruit or vegetable, as is evident from the creamy, buttery consistency of its flesh (avocado is known in some countries as "butter fruit"). Until recently, avocados had a bad reputation on account of the high fat content, but we can now appreciate their healthy, mostly unsaturated, fatty acids. These are beneficial for blood fat and cholesterol levels, which can help with weight loss and in the prevention of cardiovascular disease. Avocados also contain plenty of dietary fiber, which also has positive effects on body weight, the intestines, and the heart. Similarly, they contain a whole range of vital substances such as vitamins A, C and E, the B group, folic acid, potassium, magnesium, copper, and iron. Carotenoids and antioxidants protect against free radicals. A special combination of carbohydrates and the lecithin they contain supplies our nerves and brain cells with energy, which improves concentration as well as having an uplifting and calming effect. Consuming the fruit can produce the "happiness hormone" serotonin, as well as the "sleep hormone" melatonin, which makes it a good fruit to eat in the evening. Eating even small quantities of avocado also releases many of the nutrients from other foods (e.g. from other fruits and vegetables) so they can be used by our bodies. It is for precisely this reason that avocados are an extremely popular ingredient in smoothies.

USES

Avocados ripen after they are picked, rather than on the tree itself. So they are harvested early and ripen very well subsequently. At home, this can be speeded up by wrapping the fruit in newspaper or storing them next to apples, but not in the refrigerator. When the skin gives slightly under finger pressure, it is ready to eat. To open an avocado, cut it all round lengthways and down to the pit, then separate the two halves by twisting them in opposite directions. If you are keeping one half for later, leave the pit in. The flesh turns brown rapidly when exposed to air, so, to prevent this, brush the cut surfaces immediately with lemon or lime juice. Lightly salted, avocado is often used as a substitute for butter on bread, sliced thinly for example, or as a creamy spread. Its mild, slightly nutty flavor and creamy texture make it great for dips and salad dressing, and it even takes on a sweet flavor when made into a chocolate mousse (p. 126). The flesh should not be heated, as it produces a bitter, unpleasant taste.

CANAPÉS WITH HEMP SEEDS

MAKES 1 plate
2 tbsp (16 g) **hemp seeds**
8 tbsp (64 g) sunflower seeds
8 tbsp (64 g) sesame seeds
4 tbsp (32 g) pumpkin seeds
8 tbsp (64 g) flaxseeds,
golden if possible
2 tbsp (16 g) **chia seeds**
1 tsp (8 g) caraway
seeds, optional
1 tsp (5 g) salt
½ cup (75 g) whole spelt flour
4 tbsp (60 ml) olive oil

NUTRITIONAL VALUE per plate

kcal	kJ	Protein	Fat	Carbo-hydrate
1,950	8,140	72	145	92

1. Combine the hemp, sunflower, sesame, and pumpkin seeds in a bowl. Reserve 3–4 tablespoons of the grain mix.

2. Finely grind the flaxseeds in a food mixer. Combine them in a bowl with the chia and caraway seeds and the salt. Add the hemp seed mixture as well.

3. Add the spelt flour, olive oil, and ¾ cup (180 ml) of water, mixing it all together with a wooden spoon.

4. Pre-heat the oven to 350 °F (175 °C). Line a baking pan with wax paper, spread the dough on top, and smooth it over using a tablespoon or pastry scraper. Sprinkle the reserved grain mixture on top.

5. Bake on the middle oven shelf for 10 minutes. Remove the pan from the oven and cut the baked dough into squares or rectangles. Place the canapés back in the pan and bake for a further 20 minutes.

I like to use cottage cheese, cherry tomatoes, and freshly ground pepper as a topping for these canapés. Even without any topping, these make a delicious snack between meals. Keep them crisp by storing them in an airtight tin (they will keep for 2–3 days).

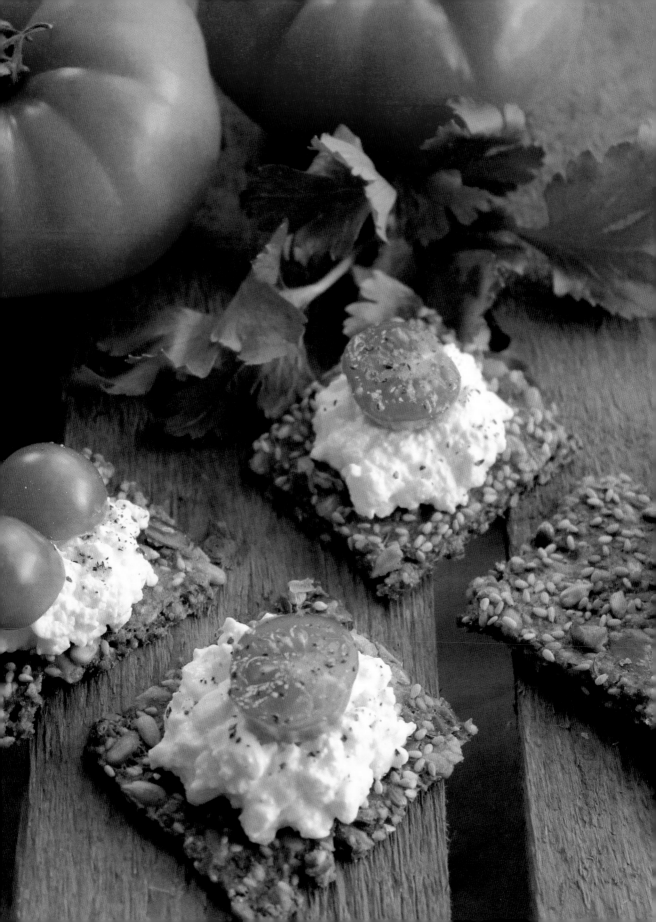

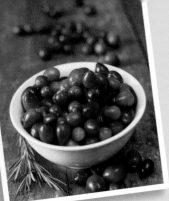

CRANBERRY

Cranberries (*Vaccinium macrocarpon*) are native to North America and closely related to lingberries and blueberries. Also known as mossberries in some regions, cranberries derive their name from their flowers' resemblance to the shape of a crane's head. These berries are grown over wide areas in the United States in particular, where they are extremely popular—Thanksgiving without cranberry sauce is unimaginable.

Like many berries, the level of ripeness determines the valuable nutrient content. Depending on the variety, the ripe fruits can be bright to dark red in color. Inside, where there are tiny seeds, the berries should be white to reddish, not still green. Cranberries from North America are available elsewhere only during the winter season; otherwise they are mostly found on the shelves in dried form.

As well as vitamins C and E and dietary fiber, cranberries contain, more importantly, a whole range of secondary plant substances (flavonoids, anthocyanins, and proanthocyanins). These have powerful antioxidant properties and boost the whole immune system. If enough of the pure juice is consumed, cranberries can also stop germs developing in the urinary tract. For this reason, they were used as a traditional household remedy for the prevention and treatment of urinary tract infections. Cranberries are also thought to strengthen the gums and protect against plaque and gum inflammation.

USES

Fresh cranberries have a very sour, tangy taste. However, the dried fruit is much sweeter, even without any added sugar. When buying them, look for unsweetened, unsulfured berries. Sometimes the dried fruit has added fruit sweeteners (e.g. pineapple juice), which is preferable to industrial sugar. The healthiest option from a clean eating perspective, however, is berries without any added sugar whatsoever. Processed products like juice, jam, and compote often contain a lot of sugar, so watch out for this on the ingredients list when buying them. Dried cranberries are a good substitute for raisins. They work well in baking (quinoa cookies, p. 136) or added to breakfast dishes (red superproats, p. 26). What's more, these sweet-and-sour berries also taste great in savory dishes (amaranth with kohlrabi and cranberry sauce, p. 92).

HEMP SEEDS

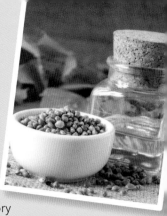

The hemp plant (*Cannabis sativa*) still gets a negative press because of its automatic association with the drug marijuana. However, the special varieties of industrial hemp that are grown and sold legally in the European Union and now some U.S. states contain below 0.2 percent tetrahydrocannabinol (THC) and this precludes the possibility of any intoxicating effect. So it makes sense to take a look at the other ingredients in this superfood: Hemp seeds, which are classed as nuts, are rich in B vitamins (especially B_1 and B_2) and vitamin E. They contain over 20 trace elements and many minerals, including iron, potassium, calcium, magnesium, zinc, and phosphorus. In addition, the seeds are packed with a large amount of antioxidants and all eight essential amino acids.

Thanks to their high content of essential fatty acids and valuable proteins, these seeds are an important source of fat and protein for vegetarians, vegans, and athletes. Their omega-3 fatty acids (including alpha-linolenic acid) strengthen the heart, brain, nerves, and immune system, as does the very rare and powerful anti-inflammatory gamma-linolenic acid (omega-6). This also corrects the hormone balance, alleviating the symptoms of conditions like premenstrual syndrome (PMS). As well as stimulating metabolism and fat metabolism, it promotes healthy hair, nails, and skin, and can reduce blood pressure. Omega-3 and omega-6 are present in hemp seeds in an ideal ratio of 1:3, which accounts for their powerful anti-inflammatory effect and is also said to be essential for healthy metabolism.

High-grade **hemp oil** is pressed from hemp seeds. In addition to alpha-linolenic acid, it contains a large amount of chlorophyll, which protects the cells and gives the oil its greenish color. Gluten-free **hemp flour** is made from the residue created during the oil-producing process ("hempseed cake"). The seeds are also made into hemp milk, which is used as plant-based milk by vegans.

USES

Hemp seeds are available either hulled or unhulled. The unhulled seeds are better suited to the clean eating concept because of their higher nutrient density. The whole seeds are a bit harder and have a nutty, slightly grassy taste; the hulled ones are similar to sunflower seeds. I use the seeds for baking (pumpkin bread, p. 42; canapés with hemp seeds, p. 52), as a salad topping, added to stir-fry vegetables, as well as in muesli and other breakfast dishes, or simply as a snack. **Hemp oil** can be added to salads, pestos, and vegetables, but it must not be heated. Like flaxseed oil (p. 67) it is cold-pressed and oxidizes quickly, so it must be stored in cool, dark conditions.

QUINOA AND CAULIFLOWER BALLS

MAKES 8

5 tbsp (60 g) white **quinoa**
9 oz (250 g) cauliflower
a few sprigs parsley
1 tbsp (8 g) caraway
or fennel seeds
scant ½ cup (100 g)
cottage cheese
2 tbsp (14 g) wholemeal
breadcrumbs
1 tbsp (8 g) sesame seeds
salt
freshly ground pepper
some olive oil

NUTRITIONAL VALUE

per portion

kcal	kJ	Protein	Fat	Carbo-hydrate
380	1,600	14	22	31

1. Rinse the quinoa well in a sieve under cold running water. Put ½ cup (120 ml) of water in a pan and bring it to a boil. Cook the quinoa in it for about 10 minutes, stirring occasionally, and then drain.

2. Remove the green leaves and stalk from the cauliflower; wash and divide it into florets. Cook them for about 10 minutes in boiling water or a steamer. Wash the parsley, pat it dry, and chop finely.

3. Pre-heat the oven to 390 °F (200 °C).

4. Crush the cauliflower in a bowl using a potato masher. Crush the caraway seeds in a mortar and pestle; add them to the cauliflower together with the quinoa, parsley, cottage cheese, breadcrumbs, salt, and pepper. Mix it all together with your hands and shape it into eight rounds about the size of a table tennis ball. Place the quinoa balls on a baking pan lined with wax paper and brush with some olive oil. Bake in the pre-heated oven for about 20 minutes.

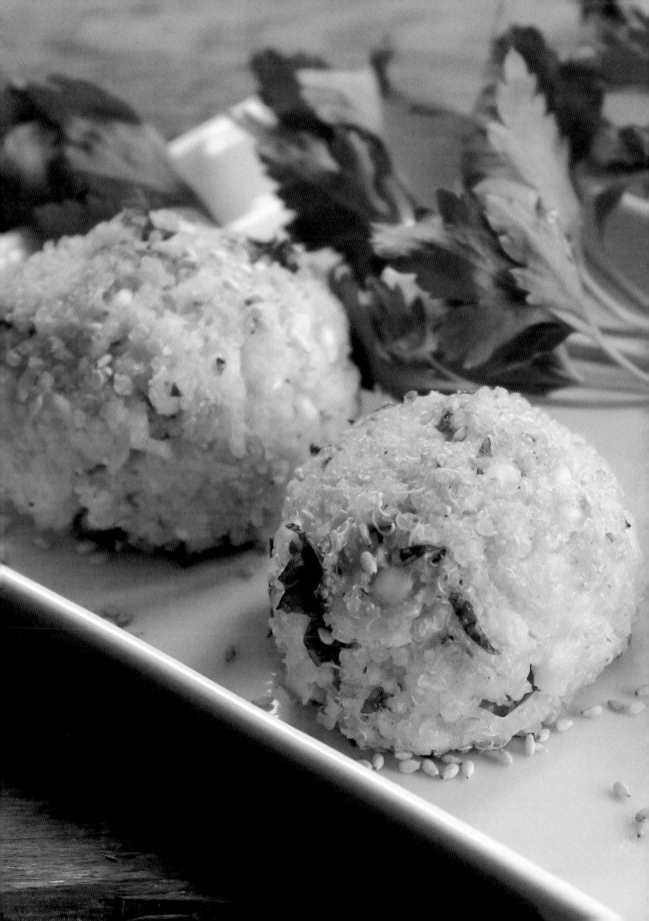

BEET SOUP

WITH ACAI

SERVES 2

11 oz (300 g) beets
1 shallot
1 tbsp (5 ml) olive oil
1¼ cups (300 ml) vegetable stock
salt
a few sprigs red basil
1 tbsp (5 g) freshly
grated horseradish
1 tbsp (7 g) **acai powder**
2 tbsp (30 g) crème fraîche
½ tsp (1 g) **acai powder**
for garnish

NUTRITIONAL VALUE

per portion

kcal	kJ	Protein	Fat	Carbo-hydrate
180	760	4	12	15

1. Peel and finely dice the beets; ideally, wear disposable rubber gloves to prevent staining. Peel and finely chop the shallot.

2. Heat the olive oil in a pan. Sweat the beets and shallot for a few minutes, stirring occasionally.

3. Deglaze with the vegetable stock, season with salt, cover, and simmer for about 15 minutes.

4. Wash the basil, pat it dry, and chop it finely. Mix it into the soup with the horseradish and acai powder, and whizz it with a blender until smooth.

5. Ladle the beet soup into two soup bowls, and garnish with crème fraîche, a few basil leaves, and acai powder.

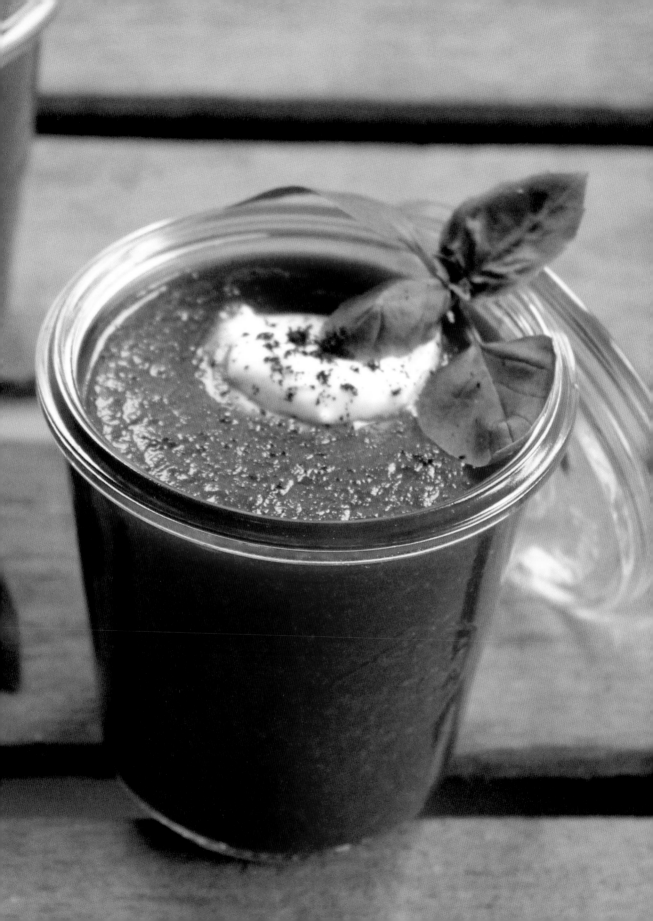

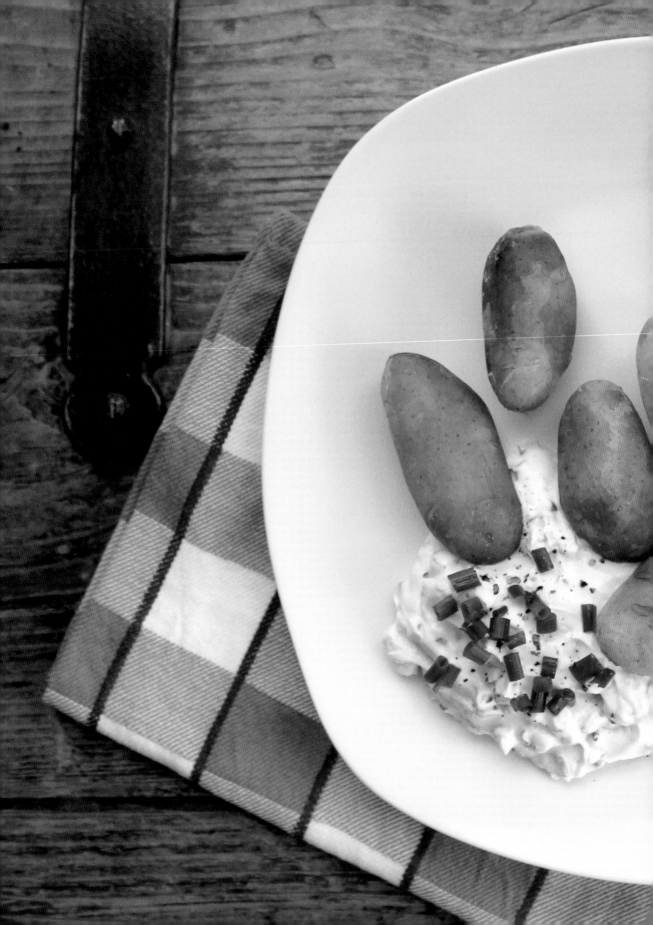

MAIN COURSES

QUINOA BURGER

WITH BROCCOLI

SERVES 6

½ cup (100 g) white **quinoa**
1 **broccoli** head (approx.
1 lb/500 g)
½ bunch flat-leaf parsley
1 egg
⅓ cup (50 g) whole spelt flour
1½ oz (40 g) Parmesan
cheese, grated
salt
freshly ground pepper
plant-based oil for frying

NUTRITIONAL VALUE

per burger

kcal	kJ	Protein	Fat	Carbo-hydrate
180	760	10	8	18

1. Rinse the quinoa well in a sieve under cold running water. Put a generous ¾ cup (200 ml) of water in a pan and bring to a boil. Cook the quinoa for about 10 minutes, stirring occasionally, and then drain.

2. Wash the broccoli, break it into florets, and cook it in boiling water or a steamer for 5 minutes until *al dente*. Leave it to cool and chop it finely. Wash the parsley, pat it dry, and chop finely.

3. Combine the quinoa, broccoli, parsley, egg, flour, Parmesan, salt, and pepper. Shape the mixture into six flat burgers with your hands.

4. Heat the oil in a fry pan and fry the burgers on both sides until golden brown.

> Wild garlic or basil dip (p. 98) goes
> well with the burgers.

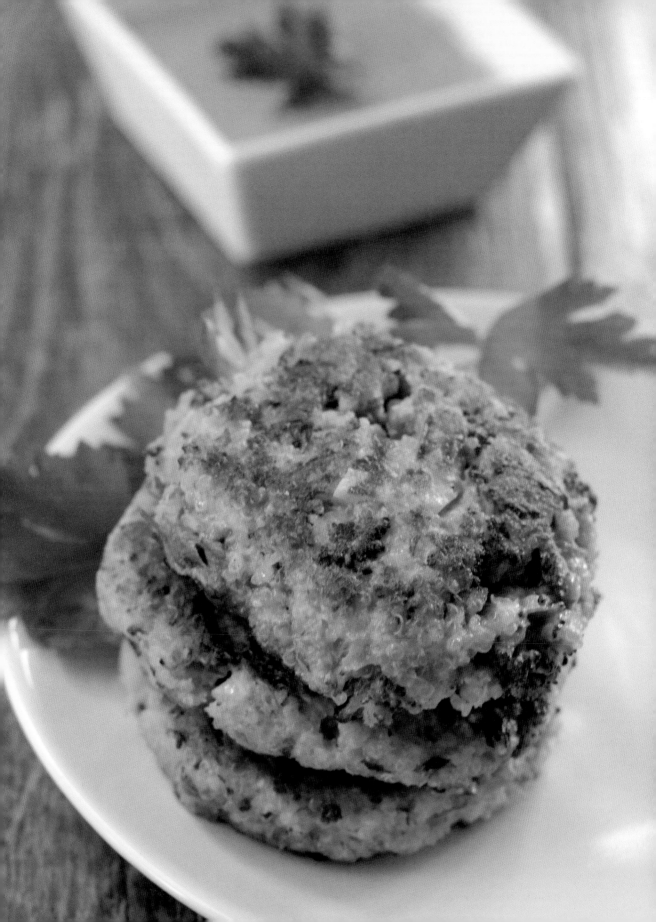

QUINOA PIZZA

WITH MUSHROOMS

MAKES pizza to fit 1 spring-form pan (10 in/26 cm diameter)
¾ cup (150 g) **white quinoa**
1 tsp (0.5 g) dried thyme
1 tsp (0.5 g) dried oregano
salt
1 tsp (5 ml) sunflower oil
7 oz (200 g) tomatoes
1 onion
1 garlic clove
1 tbsp (15 ml) olive oil
freshly ground pepper
9 oz (250 g) button mushrooms
2 tbsp (30 g) wild garlic pesto
2½ tbsp (20 g) grated cheese (e.g. Gouda)

NUTRITIONAL VALUE per pizza

kcal	kJ	Protein	Fat	Carbo-hydrate
860	3,600	36	33	103

> To make a full-size baking pan of quinoa pizza, use two-and-a-half times the amount of ingredients.

1. Rinse the quinoa well in a sieve under cold running water until the water runs clear. Put 1¼ cups (300 ml) of water in a pan and bring to a boil. Cook the quinoa for about 10 minutes, stirring occasionally, and then drain.

2. Mix ½ teaspoon of thyme and oregano and some salt through the quinoa. Whizz in a food processor or with a hand blender until it has a smooth consistency.

3. Pre-heat the oven to 390 °F (200 °C). Line the base of the spring-form pan with wax paper and brush the lower sides with sunflower oil. Put the quinoa mix in the spring-form, spreading it over the base with damp hands, then smooth it over with a spoon.

4. Bake the pizza base in the pre-heated oven for 30 minutes.

5. For the tomato sauce: Plunge the tomatoes briefly in boiling water, drain, and remove the skins. Cut off the stalks and chop up the flesh. Peel the onion and garlic; finely chop the onion and crush the garlic.

6. Heat the olive oil in a pan and sweat the onion and garlic for a few minutes. Add the tomatoes and the remainder of the thyme and oregano, along with some salt and pepper. Cover the pan and simmer for about 15–20 minutes, stirring occasionally. Add some water and adjust the seasoning if required. Trim and slice the mushrooms.

7. Take the pizza base out of the oven when cooked. Spread the tomato sauce over it, then the mushrooms, and finally the pesto. Sprinkle the cheese on top, and season with salt and pepper. Bake the pizza in the oven for another 10 minutes.

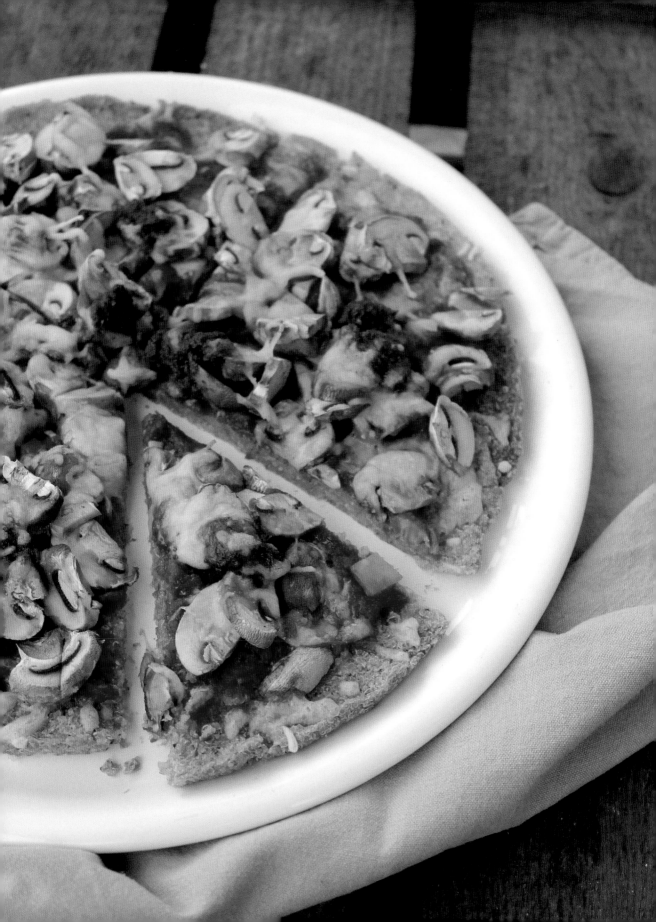

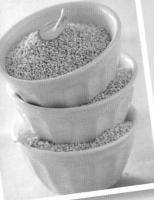

QUINOA

2013 was declared "The International Year of Quinoa" by the United Nations General Assembly and its Food and Agriculture Organization (FAO), raising the status of this ancient staple food of the Central and South American indigenous peoples ("Inca rice") once again. The intention is that it will play an important role in alleviating world hunger today. Quinoa (*Chenopodium quinoa*) is a low-maintenance and hardy plant that adapts well to different climates and is easy to cultivate. But, most importantly, this highly nutritious and very filling "pseudocereal" contains a wide range of healthy properties. During their conquest of the Inca and Aztec peoples in the 16th century, the Spaniards also recognized these benefits and banned the cultivation of quinoa in order to weaken the indigenous population. So this foodstuff, which was sacred to the indigenous people, was virtually unknown in Europe until into the 20th century, and has risen to superfood status only in recent years. And with justification, as these grains are full of goodness.

Quinoa is a valuable source of plant-based protein, making it especially important for vegetarians and vegans. It contains all eight of the essential amino acids our bodies need—which is very unusual for a vegetable foodstuff. One of these is lycin, otherwise almost exclusively found in meat and fish (see also amaranth, p. 94). Quinoa also contains lots of iron, magnesium, calcium, potassium, zinc, vitamin E, and B vitamins, as well as mainly unsaturated fatty acids. Among these is alpha-linolenic acid, an omega-3 fatty acid that is usually present only in fish (see also flaxseed oil, p. 67). In addition, the mood-enhancing "happiness hormone" serotonin is also produced by quinoa. The grains of the plant, which grows as high as 6½ ft (2 m), are white, reddish brown, or black, and gluten-free too. Incidentally, the word "quinoa" is pronounced "keen-wa," though it is often called "ki-noa" as well.

USES

Before cooking the grains, wash them well in a sieve under cold running water until there is no more foam. This removes the bitter saponins that are present in the hull: They can lead to food intolerances in babies and young children, so quinoa is recommended for children only over two years of age. The grains have a slightly nutty flavor and can be used for the most part like cereals—whether for breakfast as quinoa pudding (p. 14), as an appetizer (quinoa balls, p. 56), or as a main dish (quinoa tabbouleh, p. 68). It also works well as a salad, as well as in soup, or for burgers and patties. In baking, it can sometimes be used to replace cereal flour (pizza, p. 64; cookies, p. 136). This "Inca rice" is often simply substituted for ordinary rice as an accompaniment: Cook for about 10 minutes in double the amount of water (1:2 ratio). For muesli, yogurt, desserts, and as a baking ingredient, puffed quinoa works well, and it is easy to make your own at home (see text box, p. 34).

FLAXSEED OIL

Flaxseed oil was pressed and consumed as early as the Neolithic period. It has been virtually forgotten in recent decades, presumably due to the boom in olive oil. Before that, flaxseed oil was a popular, cheap foodstuff—and it is certainly experiencing a revival now, slowly but surely. This "liquid gold," as flaxseed oil is also called, is pressed from golden or brown flaxseeds (*Linum usitatissimum*). It is considered one of the healthiest vegetable oils on account of its nutritional composition. It contains up to 70 percent of the essential omega-3 fatty acid, alpha-linolenic acid, far more than any other vegetable oil, and substantially more than the better-known cod-liver oil. Polyunsaturated essential fatty acids must be obtained from food, as the body cannot produce them itself. Contemporary diets, however, are often low in omega-3 fatty acids, and this can easily lead to a deficiency.

Alpha-linolenic acid can inhibit inflammation, regulate blood clotting, and widen the blood vessels. It also regulates blood pressure, lowers cholesterol and blood fat levels, as well as LDL cholesterol, so it can help to prevent heart attacks, strokes, and thromboses. It boosts the whole immune system. It is also thought to have a preventive effect against diabetes and cancer, to increase mental capacity, and to alleviate depression and anxiety. Because alpha-linolenic acid is mainly found in fish, vegetarians and vegans in particular are well advised to use flaxseed oil. The fatty acid is also found (in much smaller quantities) in oils made from hempseed, soy, rapeseed, walnut, and pumpkin seed. The recommended daily amount is 1–2 tablespoons (15–30 ml); consuming large quantities is not advised.

USES

Alpha-linolenic acid may make the flaxseed oil healthy, but it is also responsible for the oil oxidizing rapidly when it comes into contact with air or light. Because it spoils very quickly, and then tastes bitter and smells unpleasant, it should always be stored well sealed in a cool dark place, ideally in the refrigerator. Its shelf life is only 2–3 months. However, it is a shame to throw away even flaxseed oil that has gone rancid; it can still be used to polish wood furniture.

The oil has a nutty, robust taste. If the flavor is too intense, you can mix it with neutral vegetable oils like sunflower oil. Flaxseed oil is not suitable for heating, so it is used for uncooked dishes, such as salad dressing (quinoa tabbouleh, p. 68), pesto, or smoothies. Flaxseed oil can add an interesting dimension to warm dishes after cooking.

QUINOA TABBOULEH
WITH POMEGRANATE

SERVES 2
scant ½ cup (100 g) white **quinoa**
generous ¾ cup (200 ml)
vegetable stock
1 **pomegranate**
½ **avocado**
2 tbsp (15 g) pistachio nuts
½ bunch parsley
1 sprig mint
1 tbsp (15 ml) **flaxseed oil**
juice of 1 **lemon**
salt, freshly ground pepper

NUTRITIONAL VALUE
per portion

kcal	kJ	Protein	Fat	Carbo-hydrate
430	1810	10	22	47

1. Rinse the quinoa well in a sieve under cold running water. Bring the vegetable stock to a boil in a pan and cook the quinoa for about 10 minutes, stirring occasionally, and then drain. Once all the water has drained off, transfer the quinoa to a salad bowl. Keep it warm, if you prefer.

2. Remove the seeds from the pomegranate (see p. 50). Peel the avocado and cut it in half lengthways. Remove the pit using a spoon, and finely dice the flesh. Finely chop the pistachios. Wash the parsley and mint, pat dry, and finely chop them. Add the pomegranate seeds, avocado, pistachios, and herbs to the quinoa.

3. Mix together the flaxseed oil and lemon juice, season with salt and pepper, and combine it with the rest of the tabbouleh salad.

> Tabbouleh (parsley salad) is traditionally made from bulgur wheat or couscous, and served cold. As neither of these grains is compatible with the clean eating concept, I prefer to use quinoa for this recipe.

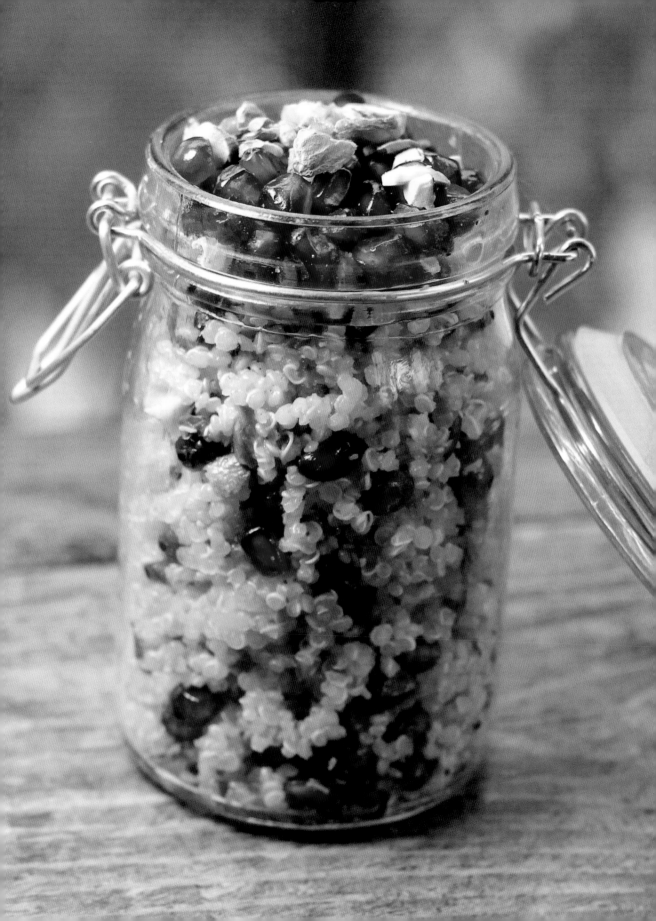

BEETS STUFFED
WITH LENTILS AND APPLESAUCE

SERVES 2

6 small beets

salt

1 small shallot

1 small carrot

1¾ oz (50 g) celeriac

3½ oz (100 g) waxy potatoes

2 tbsp (30 ml) vegetable oil

1 tsp (3 g) curry powder

approx. 7 tbsp (100 ml)
vegetable stock

3½ oz (100 g) lentil sprouts

a squeeze of **lemon juice**

freshly ground pepper

1 tart apple

3 tbsp (25 g) groundnuts, shelled

7 tbsp (100 ml) **coconut milk**

NUTRITIONAL VALUE

per portion

kcal	kJ	Protein	Fat	Carbo-hydrate
357	1,493	12	18	37

1. Peel the beets and cut a hollow out from the root ends, leaving approximately ⅕ in (50 mm) all round the edge. Simmer in salted water for about 20 minutes until cooked through.

2. Peel and finely dice the shallot, carrot, celeriac, and potatoes. Sweat the shallot, carrot, and celeriac in 1 tablespoon (15 ml) of hot oil for 1–2 minutes. Mix in the potatoes and curry powder and deglaze with the stock. Simmer gently for about 15 minutes. Rinse the sprouts, add them to the curry mix, and season to taste with salt, pepper, and lemon juice. Keep just warm on low heat.

3. For the sauce: Peel and quarter the apple, remove the core, and finely dice the quarters. Chop the groundnuts and sweat them briefly in the rest of the oil with the apple. Add the coconut milk and bring to a boil. Season to taste with salt and pepper.

4. Fill each of the drained beets with the lentil and vegetable mix, and arrange them on plates or shallow bowls. Pour the sauce over them and serve.

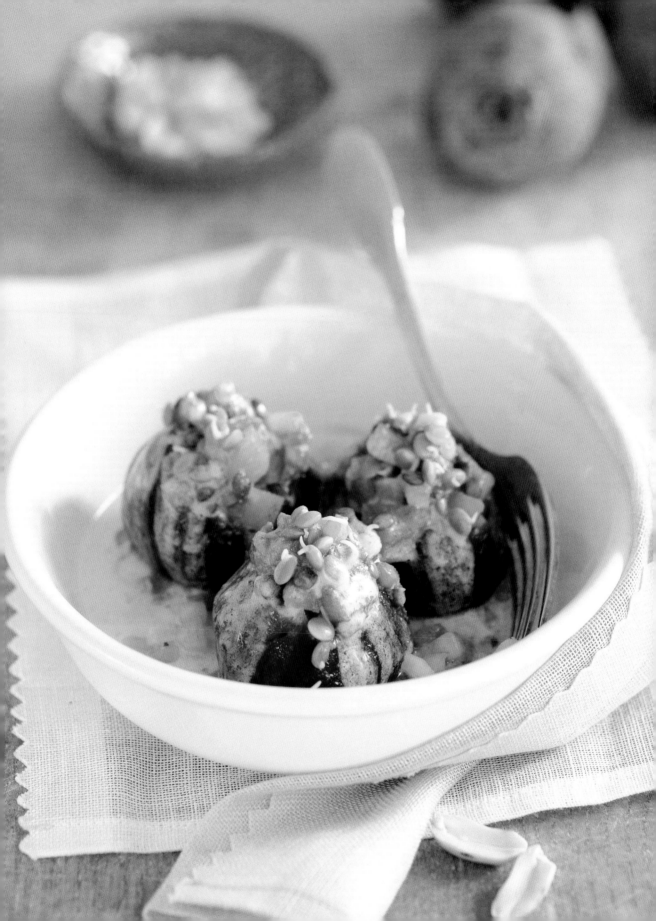

DATE SALAD

WITH PISTACHIOS

SERVES 2

3½ oz (100 g) salad leaves
(e.g. young Swiss chard)
½ cucumber
4 dates
1 tbsp (15 ml) olive oil
1 tbsp (15 g) mustard
1 tsp (5 ml) agave syrup
1 tsp (5 ml) **flaxseed oil**
salt
freshly ground pepper
7 tbsp (50 g) unsalted pistachios
½ bunch flat-leaf parsley
½ carton garden **cress** or
a handful of arugula

NUTRITIONAL VALUE

per portion

kcal	kJ	Protein	Fat	Carbo-hydrate
410	1,720	9	40	9

1. Wash and trim the salad leaves, pat them dry, and arrange them on two plates. Wash the cucumber and cut it into bite-size pieces. Cut the dates into quarters lengthways and remove the pits.

2. Heat the olive oil in a pan and fry the dates on both sides. Make the dressing by mixing together the mustard, agave syrup, and flaxseed oil. Season with salt and pepper. Combine the chopped cucumber and dressing. Arrange on top of the salad leaves along with the dates and coarsely chopped pistachios.

3. Wash the parsley and garden cress, and pat them dry. Finely chop or tear the parsley, and arrange it on top of the salad with the cress.

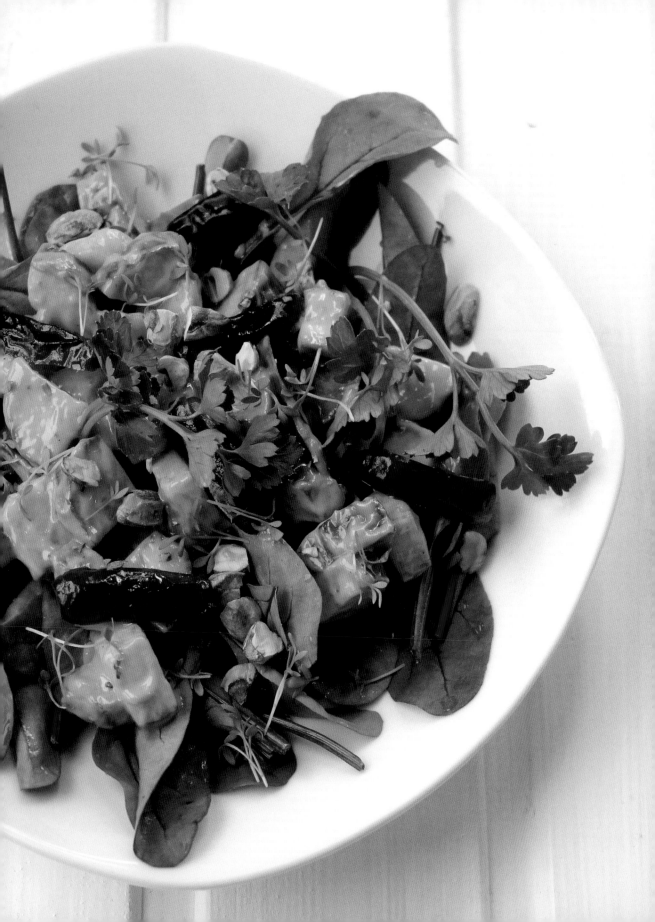

PARSNIP SOUP

WITH SPINACH FOAM

SERVES 2

4 oz (120 g) potatoes
5½ oz (150 g) parsnips
1 shallot
1 tbsp (15 ml) olive oil
2 cups (½ liter) vegetable stock
1¾ oz (50 g) **leaf spinach**
generous ¾ cup (200 ml)
cream, soy or oat
salt
freshly ground pepper
2 sprigs basil

NUTRITIONAL VALUE

per portion

kcal	kJ	Protein	Fat	Carbo-hydrate
280	1,150	5	18	22

1. Wash, peel, and finely dice the potatoes and parsnips. Peel and finely dice the shallot. Heat the olive oil in a pan and sweat the shallot. Add the diced potatoes and parsnips and fry them briefly too, stirring occasionally. Deglaze with the stock, cover the pan, and simmer for about 15 minutes. Trim and wash the spinach, then shake it dry.

2. In another pan, heat 6 tablespoons (100 ml) of cream and wilt the spinach in it for 2–3 minutes. Whizz it in a blender until smooth and frothy. Add the rest of the cream to the soup and season with salt and pepper. Whizz the soup until smooth and ladle it into two bowls. Garnish with the spinach foam, pepper, and basil.

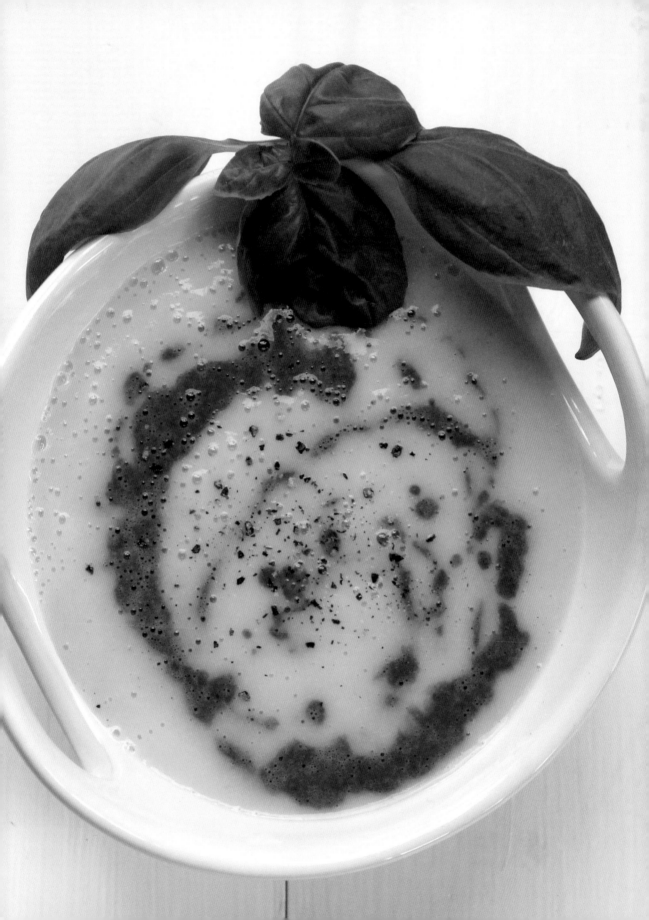

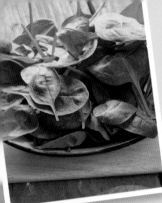

SPINACH

A punctuation error was most likely responsible for the long-held assumption that spinach (*Spinacia oleracea*) contains lots of iron and is vital for growth, bone development, and blood formation. As a result, many parents served spinach to often unappreciative children. Thanks to the cartoon character Popeye the Sailor Man, who poured spinach leaves down his throat by the canful, thereby developing superpowers, spinach sales shot up by over 30 percent around 1930. However, rather than the assumed 35 mg of iron per 3½ oz (100 g) fresh spinach, it actually contains just 3.5 mg. Yet, even setting aside this error, spinach is still very healthy indeed, a real superfood! As well as the iron content, which is still considerable, this vegetable contains vitamin C, the B vitamins, magnesium, and calcium. Dietary fiber ensures a healthy digestive system, while potassium promotes muscle and nerve functions. Beta-carotene is converted into vitamin A in the body and, along with the vitamin K content in spinach, also promotes bone development, good vision, and healthy hair.

Research by Lund University in Sweden has shown that spinach can help with losing weight. The vegetable acts like a natural appetite suppressant, rapidly giving a feeling of being full, staving off hunger pangs, and speeding up weight loss. Like Swiss chard and rhubarb, however, spinach also contains oxalic acid, which binds with minerals and thus inhibits the absorption of iron. This is usually significant, however, only if it is consumed regularly in large quantities. The nitrate content of spinach may give cause for concern, but only for individuals with kidney conditions and babies. To keep the nitrate content as low as possible, spinach should be stored only for a short time and not heated up. The oxalic acid content can be reduced by cooking, when some of it is absorbed in the cooking water. Another way of keeping the harmful effects to a minimum is to consume spinach with dairy products. This explains why milk or cream is traditionally added to spinach during cooking.

USES

Spring and summer spinach, which is more tender and delicate, is in season from March to June. The coarser winter variety is harvested from September to November. Spinach wilts down considerably when cooked, reducing its volume to about one-tenth. It can be cooked in different ways as a filling for lasagna, bakes, quiches, and soufflés (spinach soufflé with sesame crust, p. 96), pasta sauces, stews, and soups (parsnip soup with spinach foam, p. 74). It is also good eaten raw as a leaf vegetable in salads or a green smoothie, for instance.

CHICKPEAS

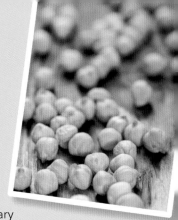

The name "chickpea" (*Cicer arietinum*) can be traced back to the Latin word for this vegetable, *cicer*; the personal surname of the great Roman orator, philosopher, and politician Cicero derives from the same word. In spite of its etymology, it is not related to peas, but belongs instead to the legume family. This extremely healthy, tasty vegetable is a staple foodstuff in many parts of the world.

This superfood is a valuable source of protein, especially for vegans and vegetarians: Chickpeas provide more protein than, say, chicken breast or beef fillet. They also contain vitamins A, C, E, the B complex, and high levels of folic acid, magnesium, manganese, iron, calcium, and zinc. Dietary fiber ensures a healthy digestive system and a long-lasting feeling of fullness. In addition, they have a whole range of antioxidants, including flavonoids. Saponins are believed to lower blood fat and thus protect the heart and circulation. Regular consumption of chickpeas has a beneficial effect on blood sugar and cholesterol levels; this is significant for diabetics, as well as for staving off hunger pangs. Their isoflavones are said to have anti-inflammatory properties. A very healthy way to eat chickpeas is in the form of sprouted seeds (see also p. 113).

USES

Chickpeas are available in preserved form all year round, either dried or precooked in cans. The dried ones must be soaked in water first, and this makes them double to treble in size: 1 tablespoon (10 g) of dried chickpeas is the equivalent of 2–3 tablespoons (25 g) of cooked ones. In their uncooked state, chickpeas contain a toxic substance called phasin, which is eliminated by cooking. So always discard the soaking water and use fresh water for boiling chickpeas. The cooking water, on the other hand, can be used as a vegan alternative to **whisked egg whites**—in recipes for macaroons, meringue, and marshmallows, among others. Simply whisk 7 tablespoons (100 ml) of the cooked chickpea water until frothy—this is the equivalent of 4 egg whites. With their nutty, mild flavor, chickpeas can be used in so many different ways, whether to make hummus, tahini, or falafels (p. 80), or as an ingredient in soups, curries, and salads. They also make a healthy clean eating snack: **Toasted chickpeas** can be nibbled between meals or sprinkled over salads. Combine 7 oz (200 g) of cooked chickpeas with 2 tablespoons (30 ml) of olive oil, ½ teaspoon of sea salt, and your favorite seasoning. Bake in a pre-heated oven at 355 °F (180 °C) for 30 minutes.

PASTA WITH CHICKPEAS

SERVES 2

6 tbsp (80 g) dried **chickpeas**
9 oz (250 g) spelt pasta
(e.g. penne)
1 onion
1 garlic clove
14 oz (400 g) tomatoes
1 pinch dried thyme
1 pinch dried oregano
1 tbsp (15 ml) olive oil
salt
freshly ground pepper

NUTRITIONAL VALUE

per portion

kcal	kJ	Protein	Fat	Carbo-hydrate
640	2,700	25	9	112

1. Soak the dried chickpeas overnight in plenty of water. Drain them in a sieve, rinse well, and put them in a pan with fresh water. Bring to a boil, cover, and simmer. Test them after 45 minutes to see whether they are cooked, then drain.

2. Cook the pasta, following the cooking time on the packet. Drain and rinse with cold water. Peel the onion and garlic, finely chop the onion, and crush the garlic. Plunge the tomatoes in boiling water briefly. Drain, remove the skins and stalk, and coarsely chop them. Whizz in a blender with ⅔ cup (150 ml) of water, and season with thyme and oregano.

3. Heat the olive oil in a pan and sweat the onion and garlic. Add the chickpeas and tomato puree, cover, and simmer for 10 minutes. Season to taste with salt and pepper. Stir in the pasta, heat the mixture up again, and serve.

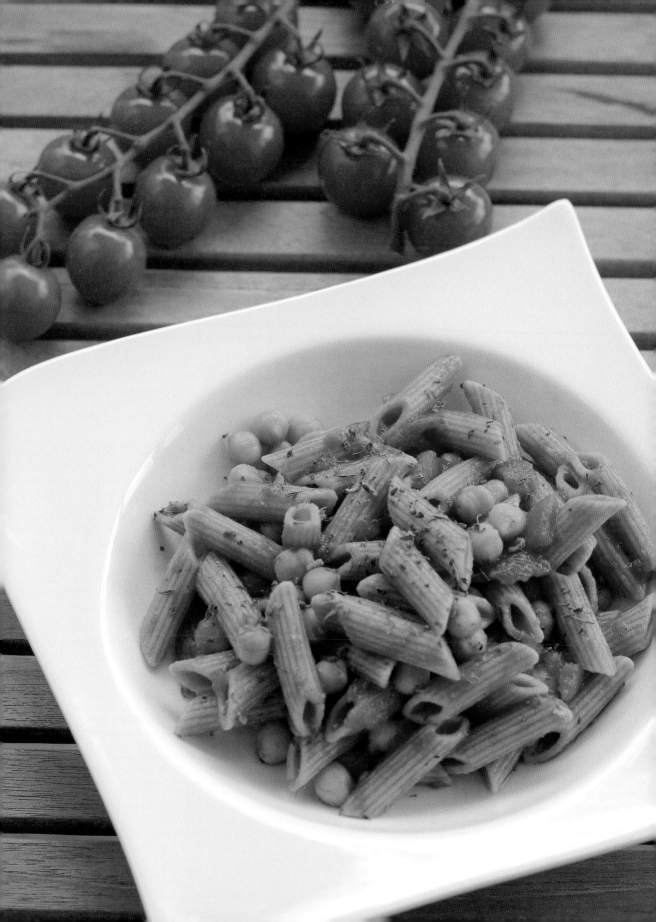

MACA FALAFEL

WITH PARSLEY SALAD

MAKES 8

6 tbsp (80 g) dried **chickpeas**
1 small onion
1 garlic clove
½ bunch flat-leaf parsley
salt
freshly ground pepper
1 tsp (3 g) caraway seeds
1 tbsp (8 g) **maca powder**
1 tsp (3 g) baking powder
oil for frying

For the parsley salad

7 oz (200 g) tomatoes
1 red onion
½ bunch flat-leaf parsley
juice of ½ **lemon**
1 tbsp (15 ml) **flaxseed oil**
4 tbsp (60 g) soy yogurt
salt
freshly ground pepper
1 tsp (2 g) caraway seeds

NUTRITIONAL VALUE

for 4 portions

kcal	kJ	Protein	Fat	Carbo-hydrate
340	1,440	13	19	29

1. Soak the chickpeas overnight in plenty of water. Transfer them to a sieve and rinse with fresh running water. Whizz them to a smooth puree with a hand blender or food mixer.

2. Peel and finely dice the onion; peel and crush the garlic clove. Wash the parsley, shake it dry, and chop finely. Add the parsley, onion, garlic, salt, pepper, caraway, maca powder, baking powder, and 3½ tablespoons (50 ml) of water to the chickpea mixture. Work it all together using your hands. If the mixture is too stiff to work into shapes, add a small amount of water. If it is too runny, mix in a little bit of whole wheat flour. Leave the mixture to rest for about 30 minutes.

3. To make the salad: Wash the tomatoes, remove the stem ends, and finely dice the flesh. Peel and finely chop the onion, and put it in a bowl with the tomatoes. Wash the parsley, pat it dry, chop finely, and add this to the bowl as well. Combine the lemon juice, flaxseed oil, yogurt, salt, pepper, and caraway seeds, and mix it all through the tomato salad.

4. Shape the chickpea mixture into little balls about the size of a table tennis ball. Heat the oil in a pan and fry the falafel all over for a few minutes until golden brown. Drain them on paper towel and serve with the parsley salad.

> Coriander, cumin, paprika, and chili all work well as a replacement for caraway in these falafels. You can also use basil, chives, or oregano in the parsley salad.

Organic Maca Powder Made without wheat grows like a turnip at high altitudes in the Andes.

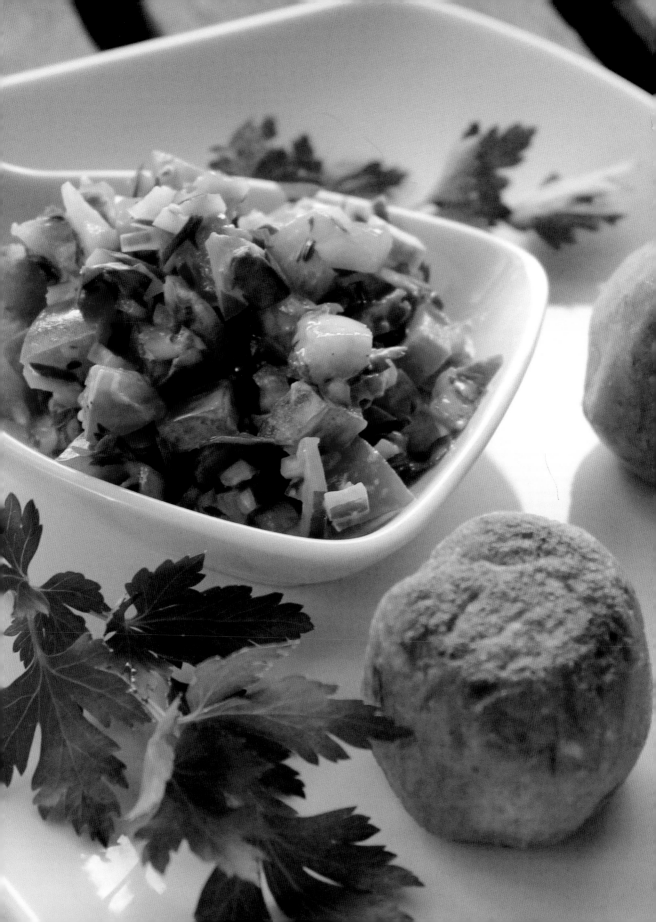

PUMPKIN SOUP

WITH CHIA

SERVES 2

generous 1 lb (500 g)
hokkaido pumpkin
1-2 carrots
1 small onion
1 tbsp (15 ml) olive oil
2 cups (500 ml) vegetable stock
salt
freshly ground pepper
1 tbsp (8 g) **chia seeds**

NUTRITIONAL VALUE

per portion

kcal	kJ	Protein	Fat	Carbo-hydrate
200	820	5	10	20

1. Wash the pumpkin, cut it in half using a sharp knife, scoop out the seeds with a spoon and discard. Weigh out the specified amount of pumpkin and dice it, leaving the skin on. Wash and trim the carrots, then slice them. Peel the onion and dice it finely.

2. Heat the olive oil in a pan, and sweat the onion. Add the pumpkin and carrots, fry them briefly, and deglaze with the stock. Cover and simmer on medium heat for about 10 minutes, stirring occasionally.

3. Whizz the soup with a hand blender until smooth and creamy, then season with salt and pepper. Stir in the chia seeds, and leave them to soak for about 10 minutes, still keeping the soup warm.

The chia seeds thicken the soup (see p. 16).

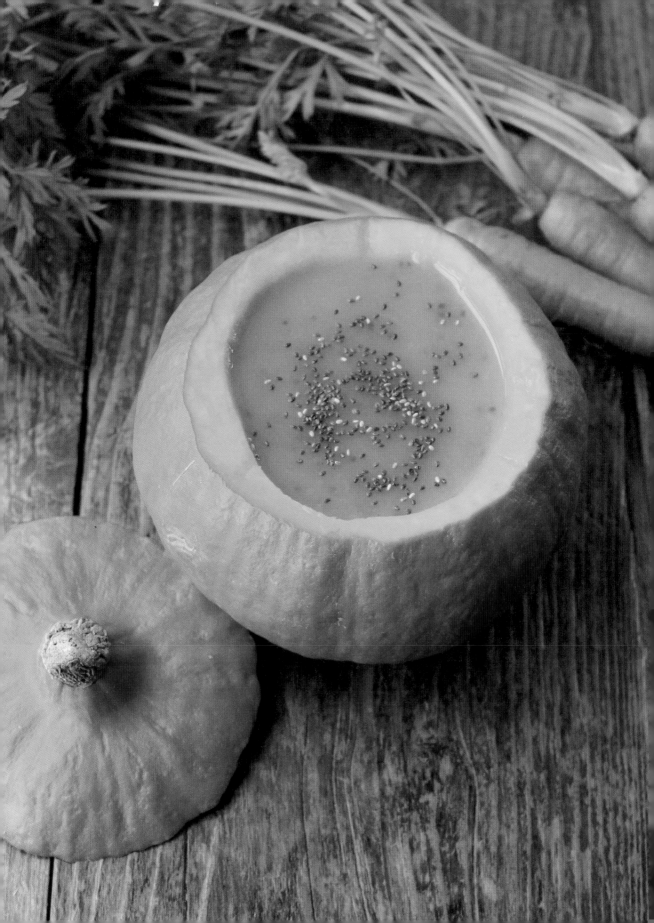

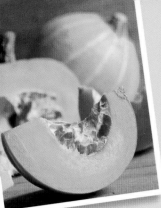

PUMPKIN

It is an old Irish custom at Halloween to hollow out and carve pumpkins (*Cucurbita pepo*) into jack-o'-lanterns. Pumpkin competitions and festivals, which involve growing the biggest pumpkin possible, have a long tradition in Ireland and the United States, and are becoming increasingly popular in other European countries. In 2014, in Ludwigsburg, Germany, for example, the heaviest pumpkin in the world was served, weighing a massive 2,323 lb (1,054 kg). Yet in botanical terms, pumpkins are actually classed as berries! There are approximately 800 different varieties in the world; one of the best known is the hokkaido (or red kuri) squash, which can be eaten skin and all. They can be round, oval, oblong, flat, or even UFO-shaped, and come in different colors and markings, often with wart-like bumps. They differ widely in flavor as well: from mild and neutral to nutty, or sweetish and fruity.

Like cucumbers and melons, pumpkin, which as a term is virtually interchangeable with squash, is made up of around 90 percent water and is very low in calories. This superfood contains highly effective antioxidants like carotenoids: As a precursor of vitamin A, beta-carotene promotes healthy vision and is important for metabolism, the skin, overall growth, and the formation of blood cells. In addition, it acts like a vaccine that can protect body cells from the damage caused by free radicals (see p. 9). Carotenoids are believed to play a protective role against cancer and cardiovascular diseases. Pumpkin also provides us with phytosterols: These are plant hormones that can be beneficial for prostate, bladder, and urinary tract conditions, and can lower cholesterol and act as an anti-inflammatory. The silicic acid present in pumpkin keeps the skin, nails, and connective tissue in good shape. Pumpkins also contain B vitamins, as well as vitamins C and E, various minerals (especially potassium and selenium) and high levels of unsaturated fatty acids. One of these is linoleic acid, an essential substance that our body needs to survive but cannot produce itself.

USES

As well as classic recipes like pumpkin soup (see p. 82), there are many delicious main dishes using pumpkin, including vegetable stir-fry, curries (p. 108), and oven-baked pumpkin. There are so many ways to prepare this vegetable: pumpkin bread with hemp seeds (p. 42), sweet-and-sour pumpkin chutney, pumpkin pudding, or the American favorite, pumpkin pie. The flesh of one particular variety named spaghetti squash can be used as an alternative to the standard durum wheat pasta. Toasted pumpkin seeds make the perfect clean eating snack, or a topping for salads and muesli. To test if a pumpkin is ripe, just tap the outside and if it sounds hollow then it is ready to use. The season for pumpkin is from fall through winter, though in many places it is widely available into the summer months as well. It can be deep-frozen, either chopped into raw chunks, blanched, or as a mash.

BROCCOLI

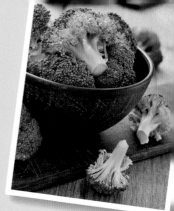

Broccoli originally comes from the Italian *brocco*, meaning "little shoot" or "little arm," which fairly accurately describes its structure of lots of little florets. It has become a popular vegetable only since the 1970s, when it began its meteoric rise. Today we expect to find it in every supermarket. Green broccoli (*Brassica oleracea*), also known as Calabrese broccoli, is a particular favorite. Less well known are the white, yellow, and purple varieties that occasionally appear in farmers' markets and specialist stores. The darker the color, the more anthocyanins and chlorophyll is present in green broccoli—antioxidants that make this vegetable a true superfood.

The antioxidant properties of beta-carotene and a mustard oil called sulforaphane also provide an additional powerful health boost. They fight free radicals, strengthen the whole immune system, and keep the heart healthy.

Sulforaphane has been found to inhibit the production of cancer cells, and research is under way into its preventive effects against Alzheimer's disease, a range of respiratory conditions, and diabetes.

Eating broccoli sprouts is also highly recommended. Broccoli contains vitamins C, E, the B complex, and the essential trace element chromium. Vitamin K and calcium strengthen bones; potassium is important for muscles, nerves, and the urinary system, as well as lowering blood pressure; and iron is needed for blood formation and the transport of oxygen through the body. To ensure the body's maximum absorption of these valuable substances, including the key compound sulforaphane, broccoli should be cooked only lightly and briefly (using the steaming method preferably), and should be well chewed.

USES

Broccoli is in season from June to November, though it is available virtually all year round in the West. The top broccoli grower worldwide is China, while California is by far the biggest producer in the United States. Broccoli should be eaten very fresh, as it quickly becomes limp and loses its valuable nutrients. The leaves and peeled stalk, which tastes a bit like green asparagus, are just as edible as the florets. Broccoli can also be eaten raw. Its pleasant, mild flavor makes broccoli a good ingredient for soups, a vegetable stir-fry, stuffing (sweet potato kumpir, p. 86), salads (asparagus salad with broccoli, p. 88), sauces, or even burgers (broccoli and quinoa burger with dip, p. 62). You can also grow sprouts from the seeds quite easily (see p. 113).

SWEET POTATO KUMPIR

WITH BROCCOLI

SERVES 2

2 sweet potatoes
1 head of **broccoli**
3½ oz (100 g) feta cheese
¾ oz (20 g) Parmesan
1 tbsp (15 g) butter
salt
freshly ground pepper

NUTRITIONAL VALUE

per portion

kcal	kJ	Protein	Fat	Carbo-hydrate
570	2,380	25	21	67

1. Pre-heat the oven to 390 °F (200 °C). Wash the sweet potatoes and prick them a few times with a fork. Place them on a baking pan lined with wax paper and bake in the oven for about 45 minutes until the skin is crispy.

2. Wash the broccoli, break it into florets, and cook for about 5 minutes in boiling water or a steamer until *al dente*.

3. Dice the feta, and grate the Parmesan. Cut the cooked sweet potatoes down the middle lengthways. Using a fork, mash the inside flesh with the butter and Parmesan.

4. Add the broccoli florets and garnish with the feta. Season with a pinch of salt and pepper to taste.

> "Kumpir" is a Turkish specialty: The insides of baked potato are mashed together with butter and cheese. Sweet potatoes make it even creamier.

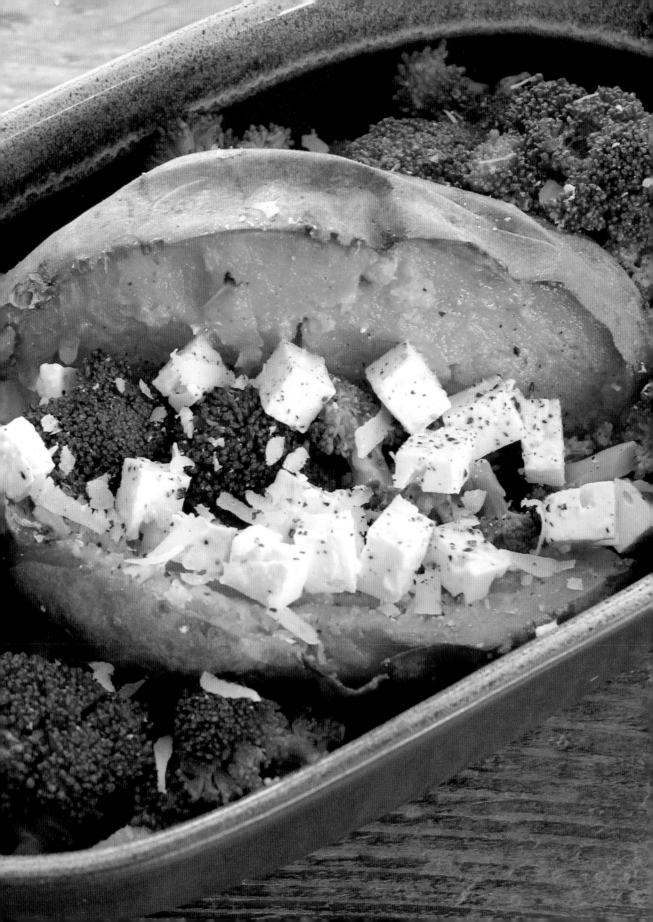

ASPARAGUS SALAD

WITH BROCCOLI

SERVES 2

1 head of **broccoli**

1 egg

generous 1 lb (500 g)
green asparagus

1 tbsp (15 ml) olive oil

2 tbsp (15 g) shelled **walnuts**

2 tbsp (15 g) shelled pecan nuts

a few sprigs flat-leaf parsley

1 tbsp (15 ml) **flaxseed oil**

salt

freshly ground pepper

NUTRITIONAL VALUE

per portion

kcal	kJ	Protein	Fat	Carbo-hydrate
380	1,610	20	28	13

1. Wash the broccoli, break it into florets, and cook for about 5 minutes in boiling water or a steamer until *al dente.*

2. Bring water to a boil in a small pan, and hard-boil the egg for 10 minutes. Drain, rinse with cold water, and peel it. Leave to cool and then slice it. Wash the asparagus, snap off the woody ends, and cut it into bite-size pieces.

3. Heat the olive oil in a pan and fry the asparagus on medium heat for about 5 minutes, turning occasionally. Coarsely chop the walnuts and pecans. Wash, pat dry, and finely chop the parsley.

4. Put the broccoli, asparagus, and egg in a bowl. Combine the flaxseed oil, salt, pepper, and parsley, and gently fold into the salad. Garnish with the chopped nuts.

> Instead of pecans, you can also use hazelnuts or sunflower seeds.

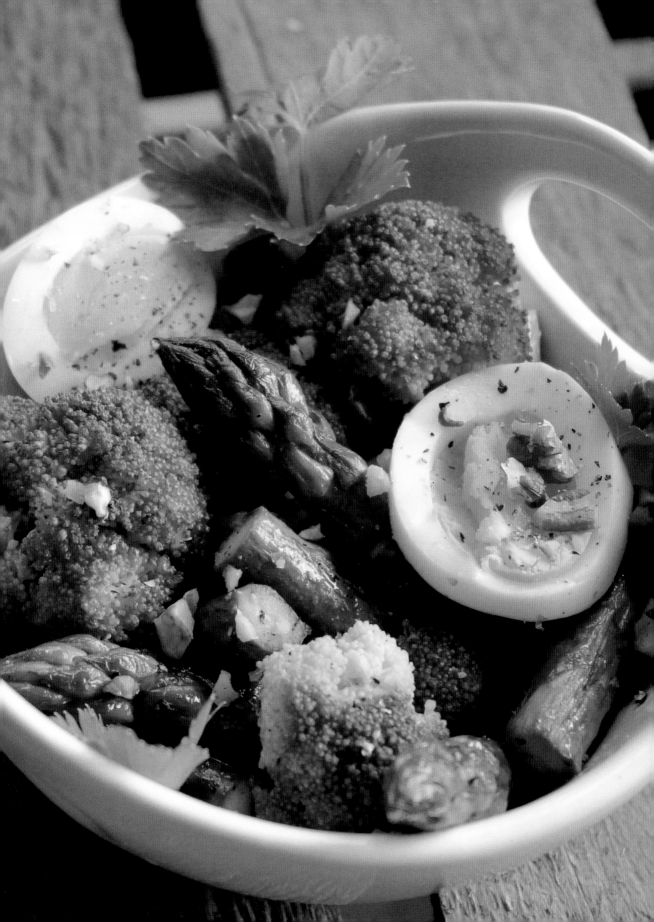

AMARANTH SALAD

WITH ASPARAGUS

SERVES 2

½ cup (100 g) **amaranth**

1¼ cups (300 ml) vegetable stock

9 oz (250 g) white asparagus

½ cucumber

2 tomatoes

2 tbsp (15 g) pine nuts

2 tbsp (30 ml) **flaxseed oil**

salt

freshly ground pepper

NUTRITIONAL VALUE

per portion

kcal	kJ	Protein	Fat	Carbo-hydrate
430	1,800	15	22	43

1. Wash the amaranth in a fine sieve under cold running water, and drain. Bring it to a boil in the vegetable stock, cover, and simmer for about 30 minutes, then drain again.

2. Peel the asparagus and snap off the woody ends. Cut the asparagus into bite-size pieces and cook in plenty of water for 15–20 minutes, then drain.

3. Wash the cucumber and tomatoes. Remove the stem ends from the tomatoes and cut into bite-size pieces along with the cucumber. Dry-roast the pine nuts in a pan until golden, stirring all the time.

4. Transfer the amaranth to a bowl with the asparagus, cucumber, and tomatoes. Pour the flaxseed oil over it, season with salt and pepper, and mix the salad well. Sprinkle with the toasted pine nuts.

> This goes well with a green salad or my canapés with hemp seeds (p. 52).

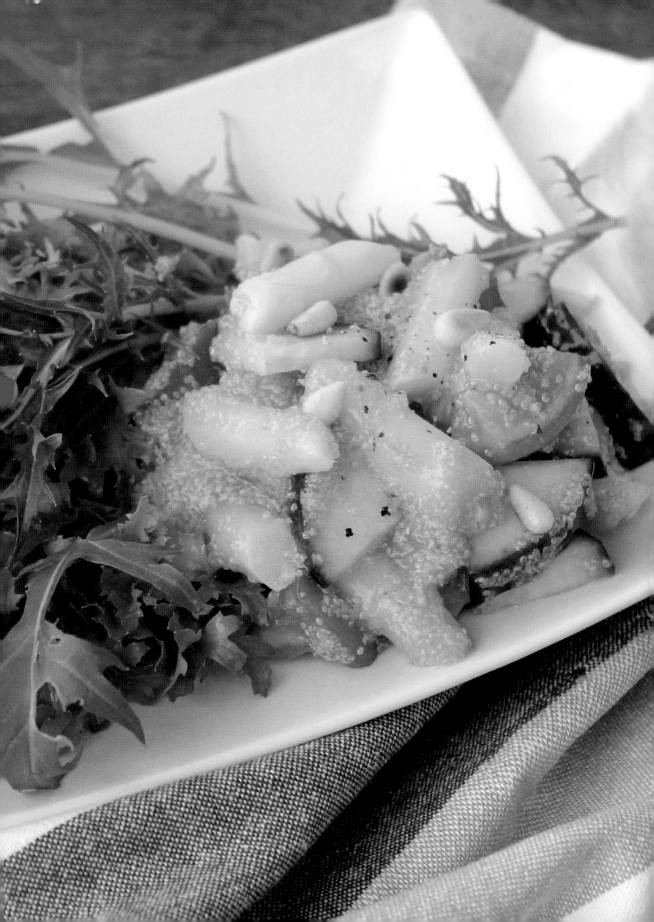

AMARANTH

WITH KOHLRABI AND CRANBERRY SAUCE

SERVES 2

⅔ cup (120 g) **amaranth**
generous 1 lb (500 g) kohlrabi
salt
1 shallot
1 tbsp (15 ml) sunflower oil
generous ¾ cup (100 g) dried
unsweetened **cranberries**
2 cups (¼ liter) cream, soy or oat
freshly ground pepper
½ bunch parsley

NUTRITIONAL VALUE

per portion

kcal	kJ	Protein	Fat	Carbo-hydrate
590	2,460	15	19	88

1. Wash the amaranth in a fine sieve under cold running water. Bring it to a boil in 1½ cups (360 ml) of water, cover, and simmer gently for about 30 minutes, then drain.

2. Peel the kohlrabi, dice it finely, and steam for about 10 minutes, adding a pinch of salt.

3. For the sauce: Peel and finely dice the shallot. Heat the sunflower oil in a pan, add the shallot and cranberries, and fry them briefly. Deglaze with the cream, bring to a boil again briefly, and then whizz the sauce with a blender until smooth. Season to taste with salt and pepper. Wash the parsley, pat it dry, chop finely, and mix it through the cooked amaranth.

4. Serve the amaranth with kohlrabi and cranberry sauce.

> If the kohlrabi leaves are still fresh, you can wash them, chop finely, and use them as seasoning.

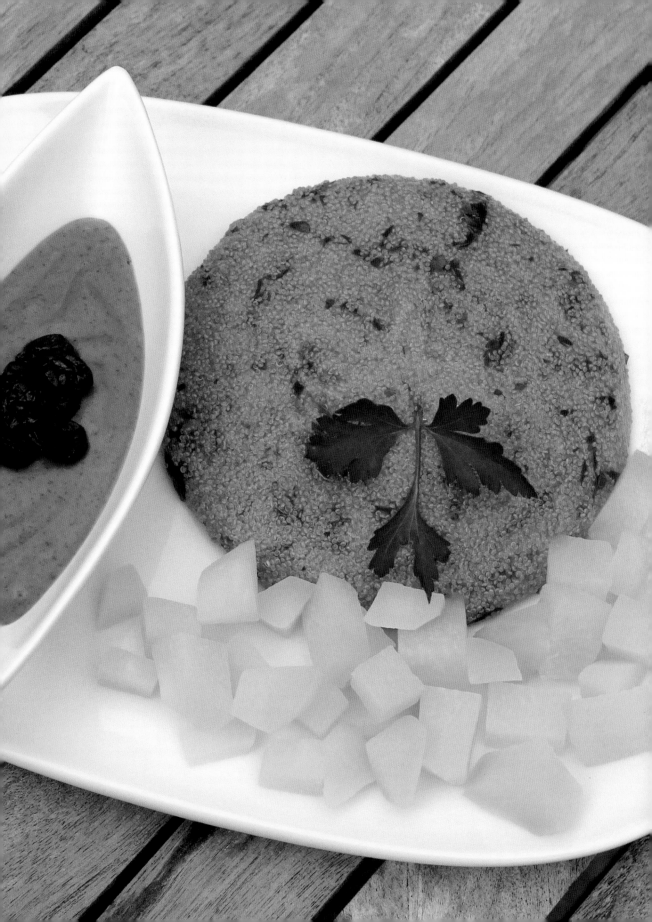

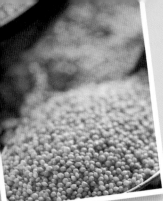

AMARANTH

Like quinoa (p. 66), amaranth (*Amaranthus caudatus*) is a so-called pseudocereal. In botanical terms, amaranthus is the collective name for a genus of perennial plants and does not belong to the true grasses like our traditional grains. We know from tomb excavations that the plant—with its flamboyant, magnificent red spikes—was cultivated in Mexico as far back as some 9,000 years ago. This makes it one of the oldest crops known to humankind. Along with quinoa and corn, amaranth was an important and sacred staple food for the Maya, Aztec, and Inca peoples. Elsewhere, this grain substitute has become more significant only in recent years. Yet amaranth's concentrated power of easily digested nutrients makes it far superior to our usual grain types. And for vegans and vegetarians it is an important foodstuff on account of its very high protein content and the amino acid lycine. It is also gluten-free.

Amaranth has all the essential amino acids that the body cannot produce itself, including lysine. Only a few (pseudo) cereals contain lysine, which is found mainly in milk products and meat. It boosts the immune system, strengthens bones, hair, and fingernails, and is good for connective tissue and skin. Amaranth also contains high levels of iron, lecithin, calcium, magnesium, zinc, and valuable unsaturated fatty acids like linoleic acid (omega-6) and alpha-linoleic acid (omega-3). In addition, it has dietary fiber that gives us a feeling of fullness and stimulates the digestive system, as well as promoting good intestinal health. Its carbohydrate content is very easily digested and ensures a prolonged feeling of being full, though the proportion is relatively low. Regular consumption of amaranth is believed to help prevent chronic headaches and migraines; added to which, the "happiness hormone" serotonin is formed in the body by amaranth. This pseudocereal is not recommended for children under age two, as it contains tannins, which could impede the absorption of nutrients in their bowels.

USES

Amaranth has a slightly nutty, mild flavor, and is available as natural seeds or flour, and in puffed form. You can easily make your own amaranth puffs in the same way as puffed quinoa (see p. 34). They taste great in muesli and on fruit salad, but you can also use them in bread, baking, savory bakes, or cereal bars. As the seeds do not contain gluten, flour made from amaranth can be used only in conjunction with other grains to make bread or cakes. I prefer to use amaranth like rice, which gives it more of a sticky consistency. I specially love the seeds with kohlrabi and cranberry sauce (p. 92), with a broccoli and almond sauce, and in salads (amaranth salad with asparagus, p. 90).

LEMON

Lemons (*Citrus limon*) are famous for their high vitamin C content: Just 7 oz (200 g) of the flesh contains about 100 mg of an adult's daily recommended amount. Vitamin C acts as an antioxidant against free radicals, so it acts as protection against cardiovascular disease and cancer. It boosts the immune system and strengthens connective tissue, bones, and teeth. This vitamin also helps the body to absorb calcium and iron from other food, making it especially important for vegans and vegetarians. Secondary plant substances, such as the flavonoids in lemons, protect our cells, slow down the aging process, and lower the risk of cancer.

A hot lemon drink is popular in fall and winter, as well as being a tried-and-tested home remedy for the prevention and treatment of colds and flu. The water should not be too hot, however, as vitamin C degrades at temperatures above 175 °F / 70 °C. Lemons are not just used in cold seasons, however: Their acidity is invigorating, so they have traditionally been used to treat springtime lethargy. Their refreshing effect is particularly appreciated in the summer months. A glass of cold water with freshly squeezed lemon juice in the morning whets the appetite and boosts resistance, while also stimulating the digestion, circulation, and fat-burning process. If you want an even bigger boost, add some chili, cayenne pepper, or ginger. As well as valuable antioxidants, this citrus fruit contains potassium, which is needed for muscle, nerve, and urinary functions. It also has calcium, magnesium, phosphorus, and iron. Lemon peel contains lots of antioxidants, especially carotenoids and flavonoids, as well as the essential oils that produce its powerful, fresh aroma.

USES

Lemon flesh has an acidic, juicy, fresh flavor and can contain a lot of seeds. If you roll the lemon back and forward a few times before squeezing, you will get more juice out of it. The juice is excellent for salad dressings—to make vinaigrette in combination with flaxseed oil, for instance. Lemon juice also makes seafood taste lovely and fresh. Try my paella (p. 102) if you prefer a vegan or vegetarian version. Lemon zest adds an aromatic citrus note to desserts and baking (nut parcels with chia and cranberries, p. 140). Lemon oil is also made from the peel, which is added in dried form to herb and fruit teas. Always choose organic lemons, as the peel in conventionally grown lemons is often loaded with pesticides.

SPINACH SOUFFLÉ

WITH HEMP SEEDS AND SESAME CRUST

SERVES 2

7 oz (200 g) **leaf spinach**
1 tbsp (15 ml) olive oil
2 eggs
1 tbsp (15 g) butter
¼ cup (35–40 g) whole spelt flour
6 tbsp (90 ml) milk
1 tbsp (8 g) **hemp seeds**, hulled
salt
freshly ground pepper
freshly grated nutmeg
some butter or oil to
grease the baking pan
2 tbsp (16 g) sesame seeds

NUTRITIONAL VALUE

per portion

kcal	kJ	Protein	Fat	Carbo-hydrate
319	1,333	16	21	16

1. Wash and trim the spinach, then shake it dry.

2. Heat the oil in a pan and fry the spinach for a few minutes, stirring occasionally. Leave it to cool, squeeze out any excess liquid with your hands, and chop it coarsely.

3. Pre-heat the oven to 430 °F (220 °C).

4. Separate the eggs. Heat the butter in a small pan. Stir in the flour, and brown it lightly. Deglaze with the milk and whisk in the egg yolks and hemp seeds.

5. Fold in the spinach and season with salt, pepper, and nutmeg. Whisk the egg white until stiff and fold it into the mixture.

6. Grease two small soufflé dishes, or one large one. Pour in the spinach mixture and sprinkle the sesame seeds on top.

7. Bake on the middle oven shelf for about 20 minutes.

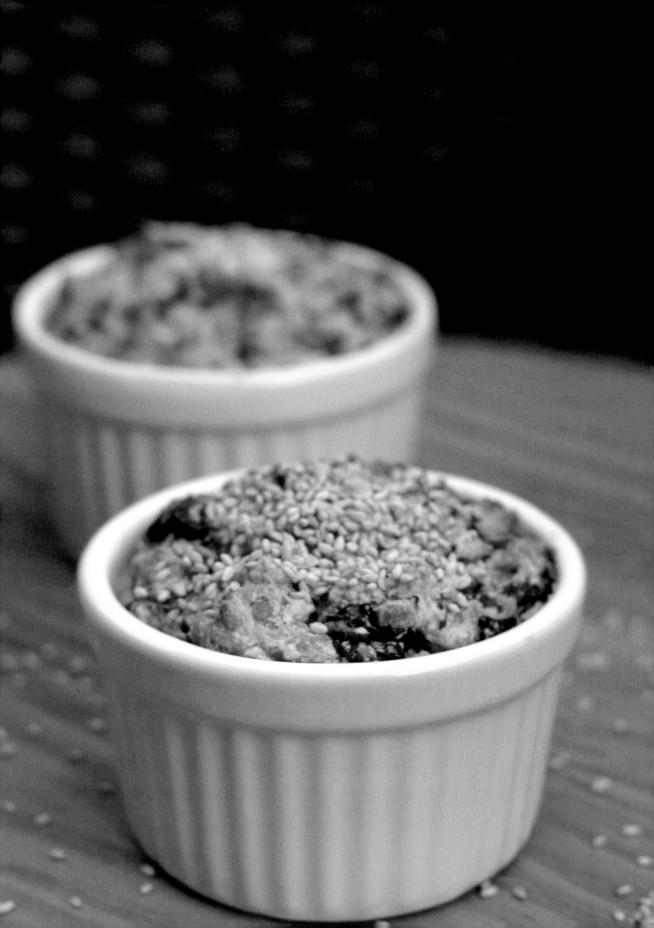

ROAST VEGETABLES

WITH LEMON AND BASIL DIPS

SERVES 2

1 beet
2 carrots
2 parsnips
4 tbsp (60 ml) olive oil
salt
freshly ground pepper
1 tbsp (2 g) dried thyme
1 tbsp (2 g) dried oregano
1 unwaxed **lemon**
2 tsp (10 ml) **flaxseed oil**
1 cup (250 g) ricotta cheese
½ bunch basil

NUTRITIONAL VALUE

per portion

kcal	kJ	Protein	Fat	Carbo-hydrate
500	2,080	22	27	39

1. Pre-heat the oven to 390 °F (200 °C). Peel the beet and cut it into strips; ideally, you should wear disposable gloves to prevent staining.

2. Wash and trim the carrots and parsnips, and cut them into strips as well. Spread them on a baking pan lined with wax paper, and brush with olive oil. Season with salt, pepper, thyme, and oregano and bake in the oven for about 30 minutes.

3a. To make the **lemon dip**: Wash the lemon under hot water and pat it dry. Grate the peel and squeeze out the juice. Mix the lemon zest and juice with 1 teaspoon (5 ml) of flaxseed oil and ½ cup (125 g) of ricotta. Season with salt and pepper, and whizz with a hand blender until smooth.

3b. To make the **basil dip**: Wash the basil, shake it dry, and chop it coarsely. Whizz to a smooth paste with ½ cup (125 g) of ricotta, 1 teaspoon (5 ml) of flaxseed oil, salt, and pepper.

Substitute wild garlic for basil for a change: Wild garlic dip also goes well with the asparagus salad with broccoli recipe (p. 88) or quinoa burgers (p. 62). Any root vegetables can be roasted in this way: Depending on the season, try turnips, potatoes, sweet potatoes, or Jerusalem artichokes.

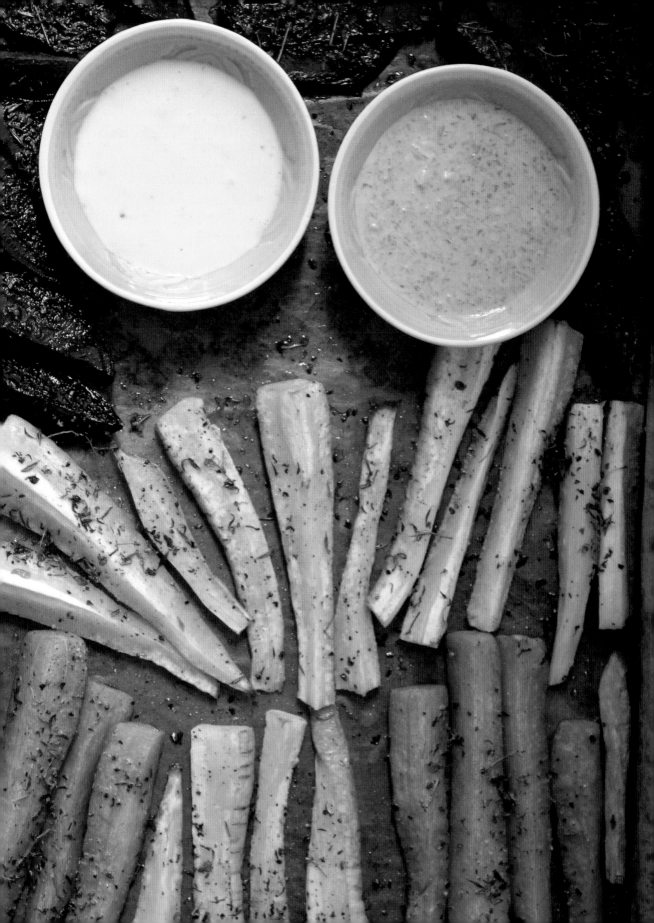

BELUGA LENTIL SALAD

SERVES 2

1 cup (240 ml) vegetable stock
6 tbsp (80 g) dried beluga lentils
1 red onion
2 tomatoes
1 **avocado**
juice of ½ **lemon**
2 tbsp (30 ml) **flaxseed oil**
1-2 sprigs mint
a few sprigs parsley
1¾ oz (50 g) dried, unsulfured
apricots, pitted
salt
freshly ground pepper

NUTRITIONAL VALUE

per portion

kcal	kJ	Protein	Fat	Carbo-hydrate
500	2,100	22	42	18

1. Bring the vegetable stock to a boil in a pan. Rinse the beluga lentils in a sieve under cold water, and then add them to the stock. Cover the pan, cook for about 30 minutes, and drain.

2. Peel and finely dice the onion. Wash and finely chop the tomatoes, removing the stem ends. Put the chopped onion and tomato in a salad bowl.

3. Slice the avocado in half lengthways, twist the halves in opposite directions, and remove the pit. Scoop out the flesh with a spoon and dice it finely. Put it in the bowl and drizzle with the lemon juice. Add the flaxseed oil.

4. Wash the mint and parsley, pat them dry, and chop finely. Chop the apricots finely as well, and add them to the bowl along with the herbs and lentils. Combine all the salad ingredients well, and season with salt and pepper.

Unlike red or yellow lentils, the beluga or mountain varieties are not hulled, so all the important nutrients are preserved.

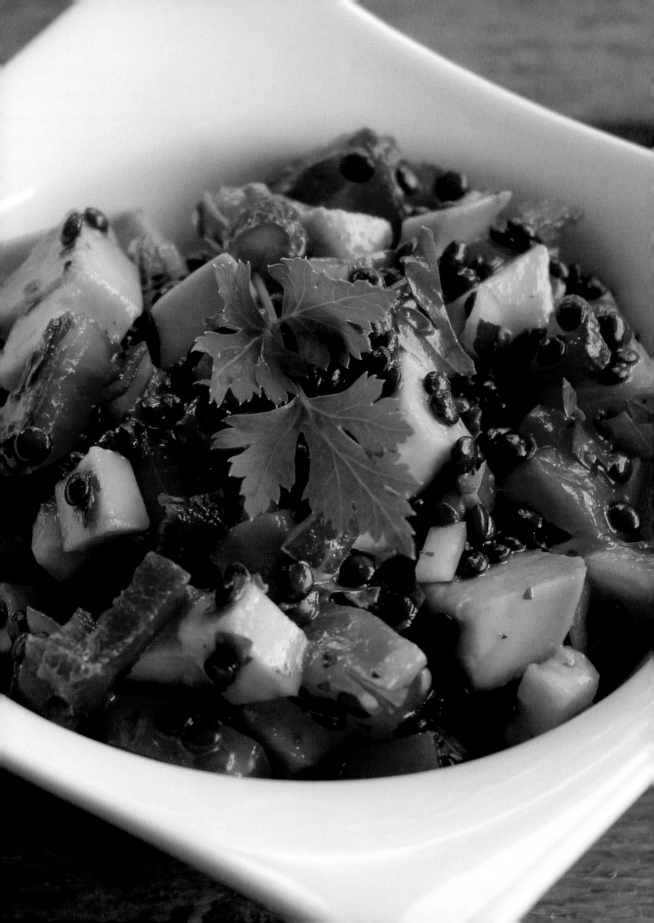

VEGAN PAELLA

SERVES 2

1⅔ cups (400 ml) vegetable stock
½ tsp saffron threads
½ cup (100 g) whole-grain rice
3½ oz (100 g) green beans
1 red bell pepper
1 tomato
1 small onion
1 garlic clove
1¾ oz (50 g) black pitted olives
2 tbsp (30 ml) olive oil
salt
freshly ground pepper
1 tsp (3 g) paprika powder
juice of 1 **lemon**

NUTRITIONAL VALUE

per portion

kcal	kJ	Protein	Fat	Carbo-hydrate
450	1,890	11	22	51

1. Bring the vegetable stock and saffron to a boil in a pan; cook the rice (follow the cooking time on the packet), and drain.

2. Wash and trim the beans, de-string if necessary, and cut them into 1-inch (2–3-cm) pieces. Put them in a pan, cover with water, and bring to a boil. Simmer for 10 minutes, or until *al dente*, and drain.

3. Wash the pepper, cut it in half, remove the stem end, seeds, and membranes, and chop it into pieces.

4. Wash the tomato, remove the stalk, and finely dice the flesh. Peel the onion and garlic. Finely chop the onion, and crush the garlic in a garlic press. Slice the olives.

5. Heat the olive oil in a (paella) pan. Fry the pepper for a few minutes, stirring occasionally. Add the onion and garlic, and sweat them briefly. Mix in the tomato, beans, and saffron rice, and heat it all up for a few minutes.

6. Season the paella to taste with salt, pepper, paprika, and lemon juice.

> Saffron, which is subtly delicious but expensive, can be replaced by 1 tablespoon (8 g) of turmeric powder. The dish will still taste like paella, and it will give the rice its typical yellow color. If you use lime instead of lemon juice, the paella will taste a bit tangier, more intense, and exotic.

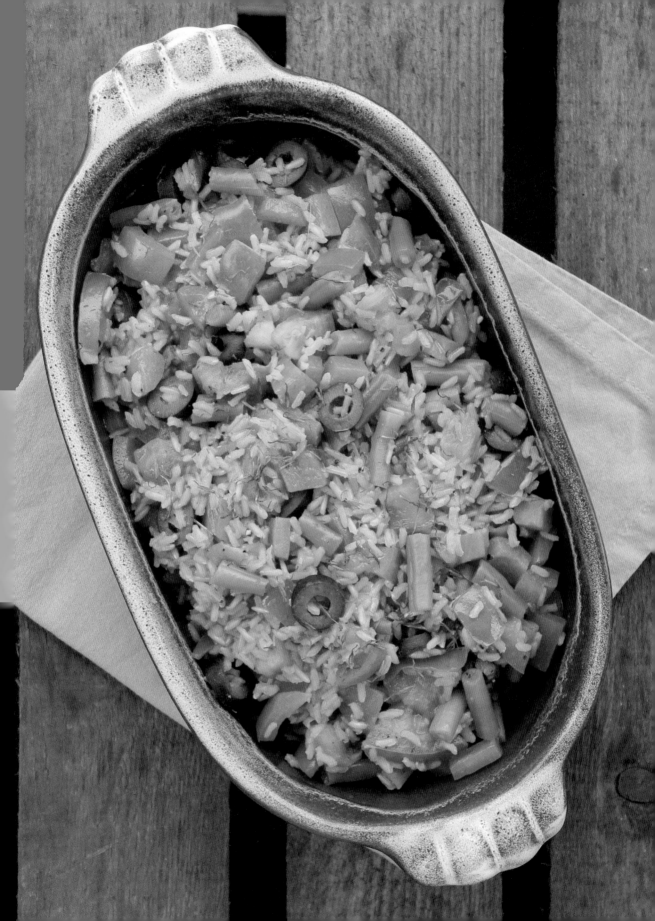

QUICK

KALE SALAD

SERVES 2

7 oz (200 g) **kale**

1 **avocado**

3½ oz (100 g) feta cheese

5½ oz (150 g) cherry tomatoes

3 tbsp (20 g) **walnut kernels**

For the dressing

3 tbsp (45 ml) groundnut

or **flaxseed oil**

1 tbsp (15 g) mustard

1 tsp (5 ml) honey

salt

freshly ground pepper

NUTRITIONAL VALUE

per portion

kcal	kJ	Protein	Fat	Carbo-hydrate
550	2,320	16	12	12

1. Remove the stalks and tough leaf veins from the kale; wash and drain the leaves, then cut or tear them into bite-size pieces.

2. For the dressing: Beat the specified ingredients with a small whisk. Using clean hands, "massage" the dressing into the kale for about 2–3 minutes until the leaves are smooth and supple. Arrange the kale on two plates.

3. Slice the avocado in half lengthways, twist the halves in opposite directions, and remove the pit. Scoop out the flesh and dice it. Dice the feta as well. Wash the cherry tomatoes, remove the stalks, and cut them in half.

4. Arrange the avocado, cherry tomatoes, feta, and walnut halves on top of the kale.

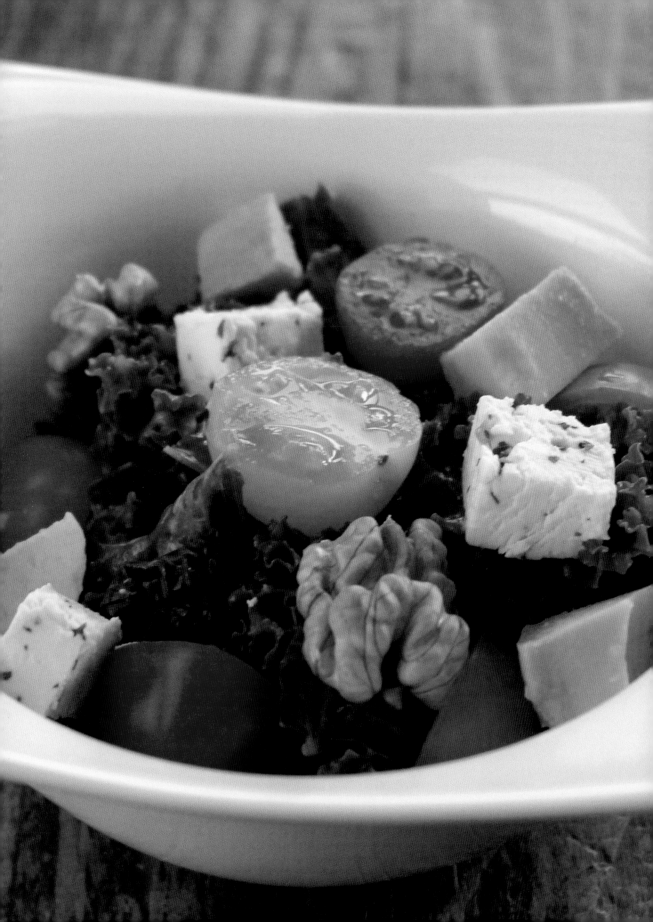

KALE

Kale (*Brassica oleracea* var. *sabellica*), also known as leaf cabbage, is a real superfood, unmatched for the diversity and density of its health-giving nutrients. Curly kale contains more vitamin K than any other vegetable: Just a handful provides one-tenth of the minimum daily requirement for this vitamin, which ensures healthy bone growth. Kale also contains well in excess of the recommended daily requirement of vitamin A (beta-carotene) and twice as much vitamin C as lemons. It also has omega-3 fatty acids, more calcium than cow's milk, and is very high in protein and iron, giving even its famous competitor in this field (beef) a run for its money! Remarkably high levels of secondary plant substances and antioxidants are also present in kale, including numerous flavonoids and carotenoids. According to recent studies, lutein and beta-carotene in particular can protect us against oxidative stress, many diseases, and even cancer. The rich source of lutein and zeaxanthin in kale also has a positive effect on eyes and vision, so combined with the high beta-carotene content, this vegetable is a top food for healthy eyes.

Kale provides us with folic acid, magnesium, potassium, and lots of chlorophyll; its dietary fiber content is also believed to lower cholesterol and blood fat levels, which in turn has a positive effect on the whole cardiovascular system. Like broccoli and other types of cabbage, kale also contains a substance named DIM (diindolylmethane), which may prevent the formation of tumors and arrest the development of cancer cells in breast, prostate, and lung cancers. This substance is also believed to be an effective treatment for hormone-related conditions such as menopause and premenstrual syndrome (PMS). Kale's rich source nutrients can keep inflammation in the body under control, boost the whole immune system, and even prevent or counteract serious illnesses.

USES

This cool-season crop is generally in season from fall through winter. For raw kale salad (p. 104), the dressing is massaged into the kale leaves for a few minutes to make it more tender and digestible. It can also be used raw in green smoothies (p. 20) or made into pesto. Of course, kale can always be steamed, boiled, or baked as well. For **crispy kale**: Wash and shake it dry. Tear the leaves into bite-size pieces and remove the tough leaf veins. Massage olive oil and salt into the leaves; spread them on a baking pan lined with wax paper, and bake in a pre-heated oven at 300 °F (150 °C) for 20 minutes. Turn the crisps over halfway through the cooking time and bake for another 10 minutes.

GINGER

Ginger (*Zingiber officinale*) is an ancient spice and medicinal plant. For thousands of years the root tuber has been used in traditional Chinese and Ayurvedic medicine to treat a whole range of diseases—and it now has a special place in our own medicine boxes and cooking pots as well. This piquant spice contains many healthy substances, including lots of vitamin C, iron, magnesium, potassium, calcium, natrium, phosphorus, many essential oils, antioxidants, and gingerol. Gingerol is a bitter compound that acts like the main active substance in aspirin: Ginger has similar analgesic and anti-inflammatory properties, so it can help to alleviate muscle pain, migraines, arthritis, and rheumatic complaints. This spicy rhizome can also be effective against viruses and bacteria, as well as abdominal cramps, nausea, bloating, and menstrual conditions. Studies have found that even cancer patients felt less nauseous during chemotherapy after eating ginger.

You can feel its warming, invigorating effect: It stimulates the metabolism and immune system, so ginger for breakfast gives a kick start to our day. You can use it in muesli, smoothies, proats (p. 26), or shakes (p. 30). Ginger can also help to lower cholesterol levels and improve fat digestion. This healing spice is a traditional remedy for colds, coughs, flu, and sore throats. Moreover, if you feel nauseous on a plane or at sea, a cup of ginger tea (see below) or chewing a piece of freshly peeled ginger can help.

USES

In tropical countries young ginger sprouts are eaten as a vegetable, perhaps an acquired taste for our Western palates. As a spice, on the other hand, it has a very aromatic to pungent flavor, releasing its beneficial properties even in small doses. Ginger root is available either fresh or dried and ground. Fresh ginger is perfect for the clean eating concept. To make ginger tea: Finely slice, or grate, a piece of fresh ginger root (about ⅕–½ in / ½–1 cm according to taste) and put it in a glass. Add hot (not boiling) water and leave to infuse for 10 minutes. To counteract the hot, spicy flavor, stir in some agave syrup or honey—children, especially, prefer the tea this way. I like the hot, spicy taste, and use ginger for all sorts of dishes, from savory to sweet. These include Asian dishes like curries (see p. 108), soups, and sweet jams or chutneys. As a seasoning, the fresh root can simply be peeled and finely chopped or grated.

COCONUT CURRY

WITH CHICKPEAS

SERVES 2

3 tbsp (40 g) dried chickpeas
1 sweet potato
½ **hokkaido pumpkin**
(approx. 9 oz/250 g)
approx. ¾ in/2 cm
fresh ginger root
2 tbsp (30 ml) **coconut oil**
1⅔ cups (400 ml) **coconut milk**
1 tsp (2-3 g) curry powder
salt
freshly ground pepper
chili threads

NUTRITIONAL VALUE

per portion

kcal	kJ	Protein	Fat	Carbo-hydrate
370	1,550	8	13	53

1. Soak the chickpeas overnight in plenty of water. Drain in a sieve, rinse well, and put in a pan with fresh water. Bring to a boil, cover, and cook for about 40 minutes, then drain.

2. Peel the sweet potato, then rinse and dice it. Wash and cut open the pumpkin, and scoop out the seeds with a spoon. Dice the pumpkin, leaving the skin on. Peel the ginger and finely chop or grate it.

3. Heat the oil in a pan. Fry the ginger, chickpeas, sweet potato, and pumpkin for a few minutes, stirring occasionally. Deglaze the vegetables with the coconut milk, cover the pan, and simmer for about 15 minutes. Season with the curry powder, salt, and pepper. Serve on two plates and garnish with chili threads.

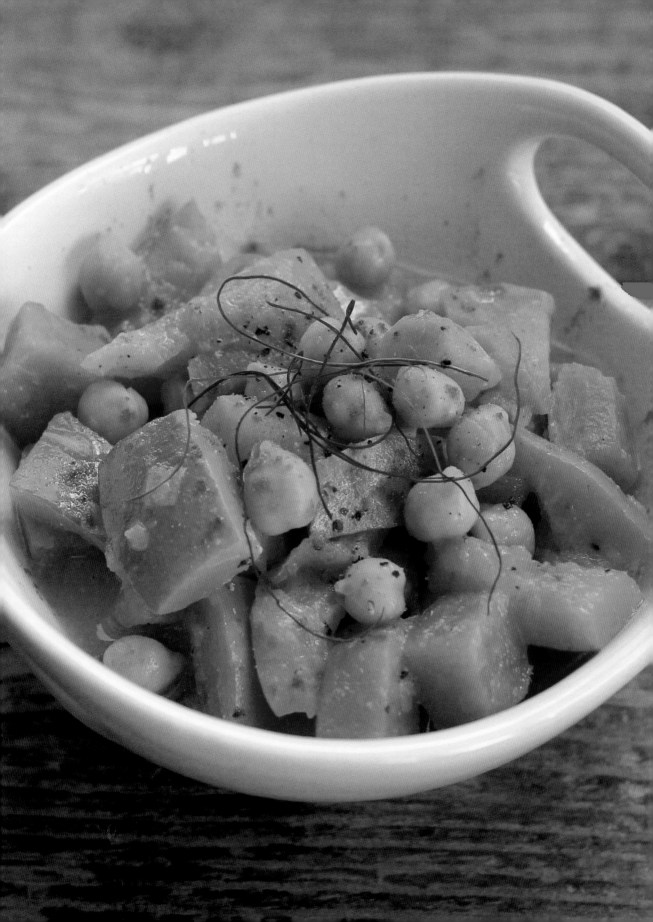

STUFFED POINTED PEPPERS
WITH WHOLE-GRAIN GREEN SPELT AND WALNUTS

SERVES 2

½ cup (100 g) whole-grain green spelt
4 red sweet pointed peppers
generous ¾ cup (60 g) shelled **walnuts**
5½ oz (150 g) feta cheese
½ bunch parsley
salt
freshly ground pepper

NUTRITIONAL VALUE

per portion

kcal	kJ	Protein	Fat	Carbo-hydrate
650	2,720	25	41	44

1. Wash the spelt. Bring a generous ¾ cup (200 ml) of water to a boil. Simmer the spelt for 30 minutes, stirring occasionally, then drain.

2. Wash the pepper and cut off the top. Remove the seeds and membranes under running water, using a knife.

3. Pre-heat the oven to 390 °F (200 °C). Coarsely chop the walnuts and finely dice the feta. Wash the parsley, pat it dry, and chop it finely.

4. Combine the spelt, feta, walnuts, and parsley in a bowl, and season with salt and pepper. Use a teaspoon to stuff the peppers with the mixture.

5. Put the stuffed peppers in a baking dish and bake on the middle oven shelf for about 15 minutes.

> This goes well with a leaf salad. Instead of two pointed peppers, you can also use two ordinary bell peppers; and fresh basil makes a good substitute for parsley.

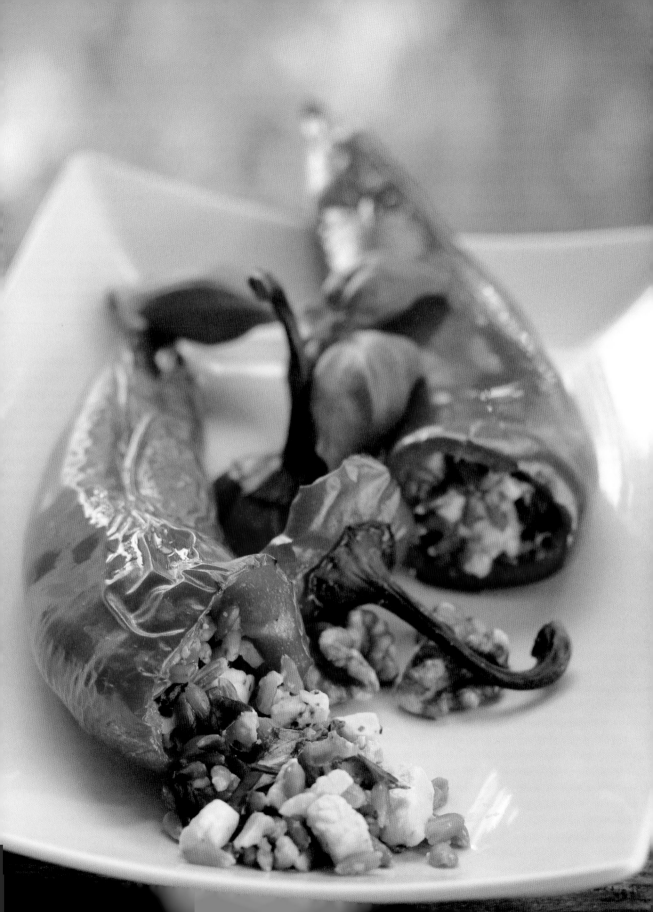

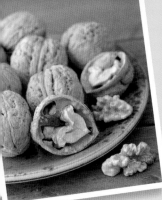

WALNUTS

As well as resembling a human brain, walnuts are indeed a real "brain food." Just as the skull shields our brain, the walnut's hard, light-brown shell protects it from damage, when the nut falls from the tree for instance. Walnut trees (*Juglans regia*) may take 10 to 20 years to bear fruit, but thereafter they churn out as much as 330 lb (150 kg) of nuts per year. Although the season is short, walnuts in their shells stay fresh for about a year. So they are available all year round, which is fortunate for us. Walnuts are rightly reputed to be good for the nervous system, as they improve our concentration and performance. Walnuts contain almost twice as many antioxidants as other nuts, which makes them not just a brain food, but a superfood as well.

Eaten regularly, the flavonoids and other antioxidants in walnuts increase our mental capacity and memory, and are believed to delay and alleviate the onset of Alzheimer's.

The kernels contain some 15 percent protein and 60 percent fat. The mono and polyunsaturated fatty acids include alpha-linoleic acid, an essential omega-3 fatty acid that our body cannot produce itself. It is important for the development of the brain and nerve cells, and prevents among other things cardiovascular disease (see also flaxseed oil, p. 67). Blood fat, cholesterol, and unhealthy LDL cholesterol values can all be lowered by eating walnuts on a regular basis. In addition, walnuts are rich in zinc, lecithin, magnesium, iron, phosphorus, calcium, and potassium, and they contain vitamins A, C, E, and the B complex. According to research by Pennsylvania State University, nine walnuts plus 1 teaspoon of walnut oil per day protects against high blood pressure caused by stress. Combining it with flaxseed oil showed an improvement in arterial health. By eating a fairly small portion of walnuts each day, we can improve our blood sugar levels, and so protect ourselves against type 2 diabetes.

USES

Walnuts are a very versatile ingredient and a healthy clean eating snack for between meals. You can have them chopped as a topping for bakes or salads (Waldorf salad, p. 114); in a vinaigrette in the form of walnut oil; or in baking. Their mild, nutty flavor goes just as well in savory breads (khorasan and walnut rolls, p. 40; bread with nuts and berries, p. 12) as in sweet baked goods like walnut brownies (p. 130). They should be used quickly if shelled and chopped, as they soon turn rancid. So it is best to crack them fresh, and eat a handful now and again. The very hard nuts open quite easily if left in the freezer for an hour.

SPROUTS

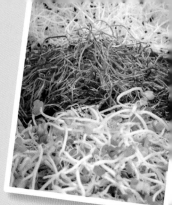

Sprouts are food in its pure, unadulterated form, so this makes them the ultimate in clean eating. The vitamin content of seeds increases considerably during germination; this applies to vitamins C, E, and K, beta-carotene (provitamin A), and the important B vitamins. Vitamin B_{12} has also been found in some pulse sprouts, a vitamin usually present only in animal products and sauerkraut. Sprouts also provide calcium, magnesium, potassium, phosphorus, and zinc, as well as high-grade protein and lots of antioxidants. The germination process makes their carbohydrate content more digestible. Scientists at the University Hospital in Heidelberg, Germany have recently found in laboratory tests that broccoli sprouts have a cancer-inhibiting effect.

Sprouts can be grown quite easily from just about any seed sown at home: from grains (e.g. wheat, oats, spelt, khorasan), pseudocereals (amaranth, quinoa), pulses (alfalfa, peas, mung beans, small garden beans), root vegetables (radish, beets), brassicas (broccoli), or spices (fennel, aniseed, caraway). The germination period ranges from 2 to 8 days, depending on the variety. All sprouts can be eaten raw, except peas, chickpeas, and adzuki beans, which must be heated for several minutes to neutralize the toxic phasin in them. Sprouts must be washed very well before eating and used within 2-3 days. Mold can form if there is waterlogging, too little water, or incorrect temperatures or light conditions. The thin, healthy fibrous roots of the sprouts can easily be mistaken, however, for mold, which has a very musty, acrid smell. Any moldy sprouts must be immediately discarded. More and more supermarkets are stocking ready-to-eat sprouts in the chiller section. Food hygiene agencies recommend that prepacked sprouts should be consumed as soon as possible; and, following an *E. coli* outbreak in Germany in 2011, the advice for people with weakened immune systems is to avoid them completely. Sprouts were officially identified as the likely source of the outbreak, which has tarnished their image to a great extent.

USES

All sprouts have a lovely, fresh, and crispy taste. Their flavors range from sweetish (grains like wheat and oats), through mild to nutty (lentils, alfalfa, chickpeas), to refreshingly robust (broccoli), slightly spicy (cress, arugula), and very peppery (various types of radish). Sprouts are used as a topping for salads and soups, or served in wraps and sandwiches. They also taste good in sweet dishes like muesli, yogurt, and desserts (p. 124). Or you can add them to omelets, stir-fries, pasta, and rice dishes—a burst of freshness for just about any dish!

WALDORF SALAD

SERVES 2

9 oz (250 g) celeriac
juice of ½ **lemon**
1 apple
10 tbsp (150 g) soy or
other natural yogurt
salt
freshly ground pepper
¼ cup (30 g) shelled **walnuts**

NUTRITIONAL VALUE

per portion

kcal	kJ	Protein	Fat	Carbo-hydrate
230	950	8	14	17

1. Trim and peel the celeriac. Grate it coarsely, or cut it into very thin bite-size strips with a julienne peeler. Combine it immediately with the lemon juice in a salad bowl to prevent it turning brown.

2. Wash and quarter the apple, and remove the stalk and core. Chop it finely too, and mix it well through the celeriac. Add the yogurt, salt and pepper, mix well, and let it soak for a few minutes.

3. Finely chop the shelled walnuts and sprinkle them over the salad.

Classic Waldorf salad contains a lot of mayonnaise, which is incompatible with the clean eating concept. Yogurt makes the salad much lighter and vegan, if you use soy yogurt. If you like, add more seasoning in the form of curry or chili; grapes or pomegranate also work well.

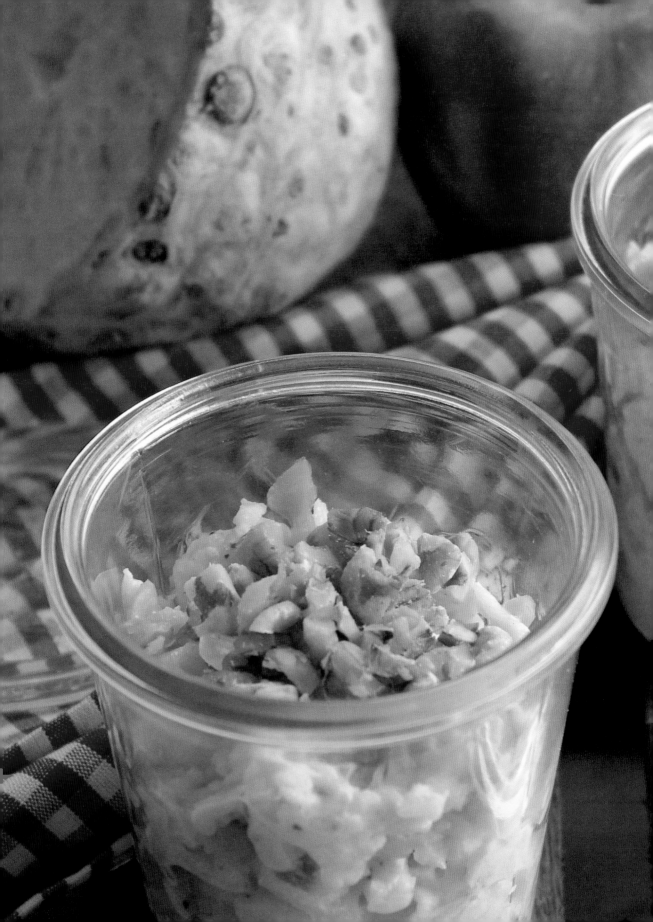

FRUITY

BEET SALAD

SERVES 2

1 beet (approx. 7 oz/200 g)
3½ oz (100 g) arugula
1 apple
2 tbsp (15 g) shelled **walnuts**
2 tbsp (15 g) pecan nuts
2 tbsp (30 ml) **walnut oil**
salt
freshly ground pepper

NUTRITIONAL VALUE

per portion

kcal	kJ	Protein	Fat	Carbo-hydrate
330	1,360	6	25	20

1. Peel the beet, cut it in half, and then into slices about ⅕ in (½ cm) thick; ideally, use disposable gloves to avoid staining. Steam the beet slices for about 15 minutes until *al dente.*

2. Wash and trim the arugula, then shake it dry. Wash and quarter the apple, remove the core, and slice it thinly. Coarsely chop the nuts.

3. Divide the arugula between two plates. Arrange the beet, apple, and nuts on top. Drizzle the walnut oil over the salad and season with salt and pepper.

> This goes well with quinoa balls (p. 56) or the spinach soufflé with sesame crust (p. 96).

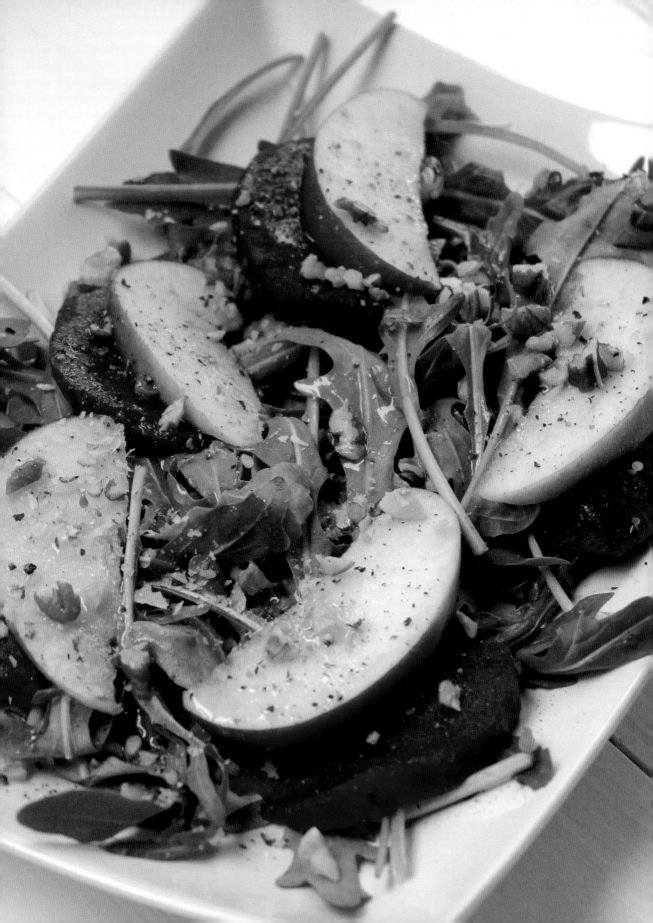

KALE AND RICE STIR-FRY

SERVES 2

½ cup (100 g) whole-grain rice
11 oz (300 g) **kale**
1 onion
2 tbsp (30 ml) olive oil
salt
freshly ground pepper
2 tbsp (16 g) **hemp seeds**

NUTRITIONAL VALUE

per portion

kcal	kJ	Protein	Fat	Carbo-hydrate
350	1,470	12	14	43

1. Cook the rice (follow the cooking times on the packet). Remove the stalks and tough leaf veins from the kale, and wash the leaves.

2. Bring water to a boil in a pan and blanch the kale for 3–5 minutes. Drain well, and squeeze out any excess moisture. Chop the leaves very finely.

3. Peel and finely dice the onion. Heat the olive oil in a pan and fry the onion. Add the whole-grain rice and kale, and fry for about 5 minutes, stirring occasionally. Season with salt and pepper, and arrange on two plates (see text box). Garnish with the hemp seeds.

> To make the rice dish look more appetizing, use a serving ring or a cup greased lightly with oil. Fill it with the rice mixture and press it down with a spoon. Turn it onto a plate—job done.

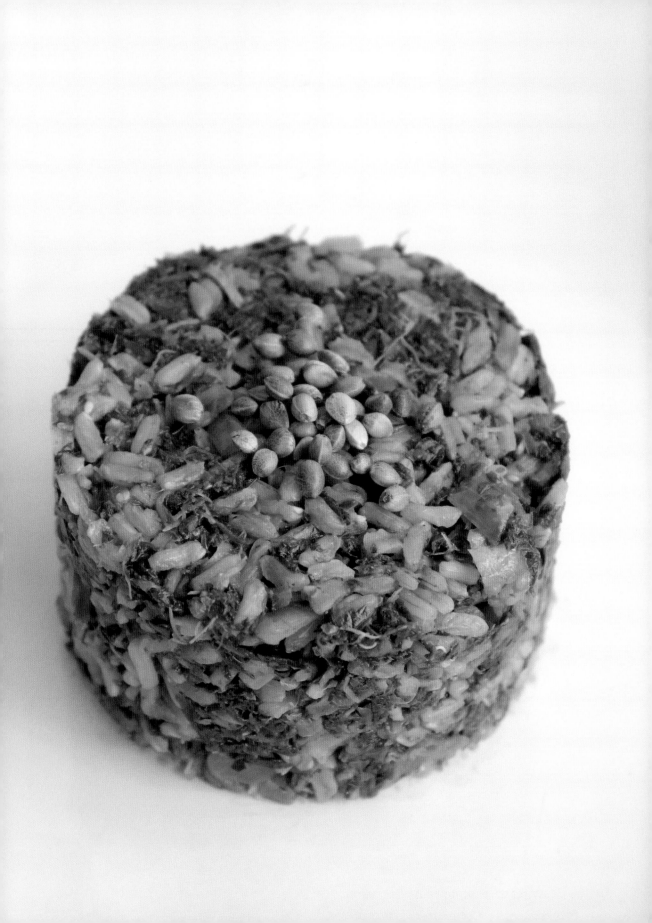

POTATO WEDGES

WITH ASPARAGUS AND VEGETABLE SAUCE

SERVES 2

generous 1 lb (500 g) potatoes
generous 1 lb (500 g)
green asparagus
2 tbsp (30 ml) olive oil
salt
freshly ground pepper
2 tbsp **sprouts**
(e.g. radishes, alfalfa,
mung beans)

For the sauce

1 shallot
1 garlic clove
2 oz (60 g) potato
1 oz (30 g) carrot
1 tbsp (15 g) butter or margarine
¼ cup (30 g) cashew
nuts or 2-3 tbsp
cashew or almond butter
salt
freshly ground pepper

NUTRITIONAL VALUE

per portion

kcal	kJ	Protein	Fat	Carbo-hydrate
480	2,010	14	22	55

1. Pre-heat the oven to 355 °F (180 °C). Wash the potatoes and cut them lengthways into eight wedges. Wash the asparagus and snap off the woody ends. Place the potatoes and asparagus on a baking pan lined with wax paper and brush with olive oil. Season with salt and pepper. Bake on the middle oven shelf for about 30 minutes, turning halfway through.

2. To make the vegetable sauce: Peel and finely dice the shallot. Peel and crush the garlic. Peel the potato and carrot, and chop them into small pieces.

3. Heat the butter in a pan, and sweat the onion and garlic. Add the potato and carrot, and fry them briefly as well. Deglaze with 7 tablespoons (100 ml) of water and add the cashew nuts. Simmer gently for 15 minutes, stirring from time to time. Season with salt and pepper, and whizz the sauce in a blender until smooth.

4. Arrange the potato wedges and asparagus on two plates, coat with the sauce, and garnish with the sprouts.

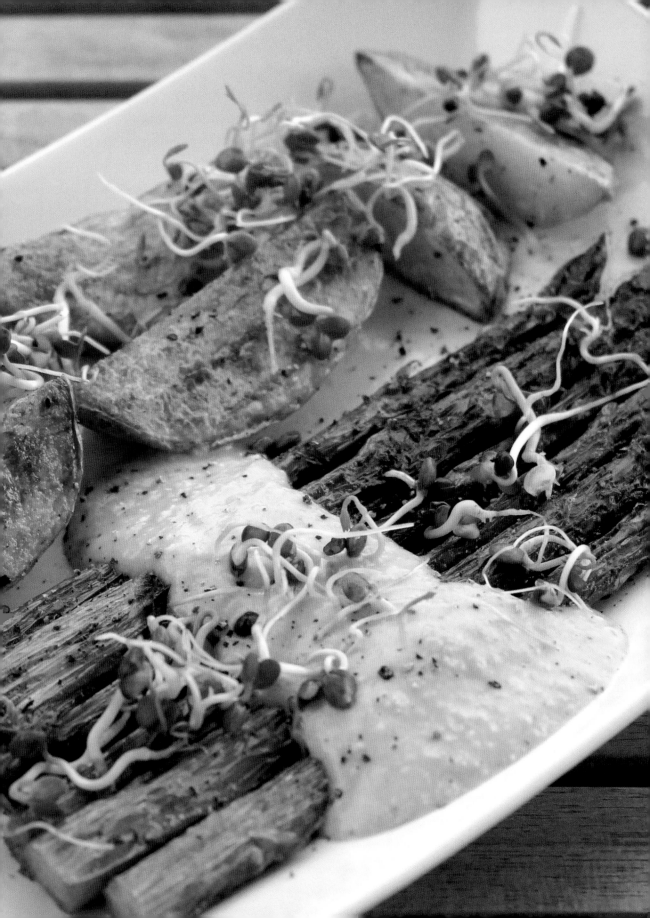

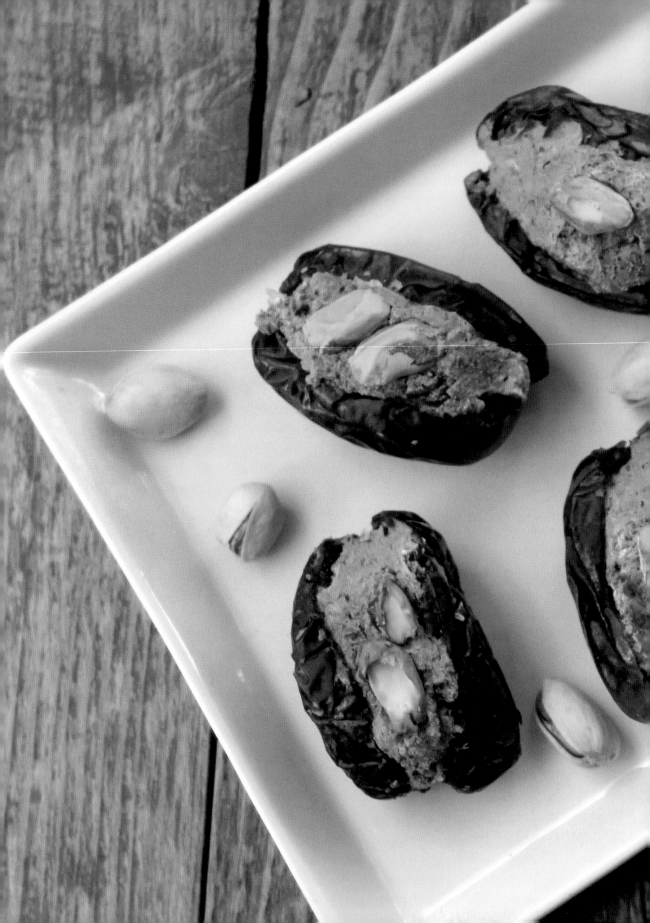

DESSERTS
& CAKES

PINEAPPLE CARPACCIO

WITH MINT SAUCE AND COCOA NIBS

SERVES 2
½ pineapple
2 sprigs mint
1 lime
2 tbsp (16 g) **cocoa nibs**

NUTRITIONAL VALUE

per portion

kcal	kJ	Protein	Fat	Carbo-hydrate
190	770	2	2	37

1. Cut off the top and bottom ends of the pineapple. Stand it upright and slice off the skin and all the brown bits ("eyes").

2. Cut off wafer-thin slices of pineapple flesh, and remove the hard central core. Arrange the slices on two plates.

3. Wash the mint, pat it dry, and cut it into thin strips. Squeeze the juice from the lime and combine it with the mint. Drizzle the mint sauce over the sliced pineapple and garnish with cocoa nibs.

> Instead of nibs, you can also use other superfoods like goji berries, cranberries, or hulled hemp seeds.

PEACHES

STUFFED WITH SPROUTS

SERVES 2
2 peaches
⅓ cup (80 g) ricotta cheese
½ tsp (2 g) Ceylon cinnamon powder
½ tsp (2 g) **carob powder**
1 tbsp (8 g) **cocoa nibs**
¼ cup (25 g) **sprouts**
(e.g. mung beans, radishes, wheat)
some **cocoa nibs** for garnish

NUTRITIONAL VALUE

per portion

kcal	kJ	Protein	Fat	Carbohy-drate.
200	830	6	11	18

1. Wash the peach, pat it dry, cut in half, and remove the pit.

2. Combine the ricotta, cinnamon, carob powder, and cocoa nibs; divide the mixture between the peach halves.

3. Garnish with sprouts and cocoa nibs.

> Instead of carob powder, you can also use raw cocoa powder. And if you want to omit the cinnamon, just increase the amount of carob or cocoa powder.

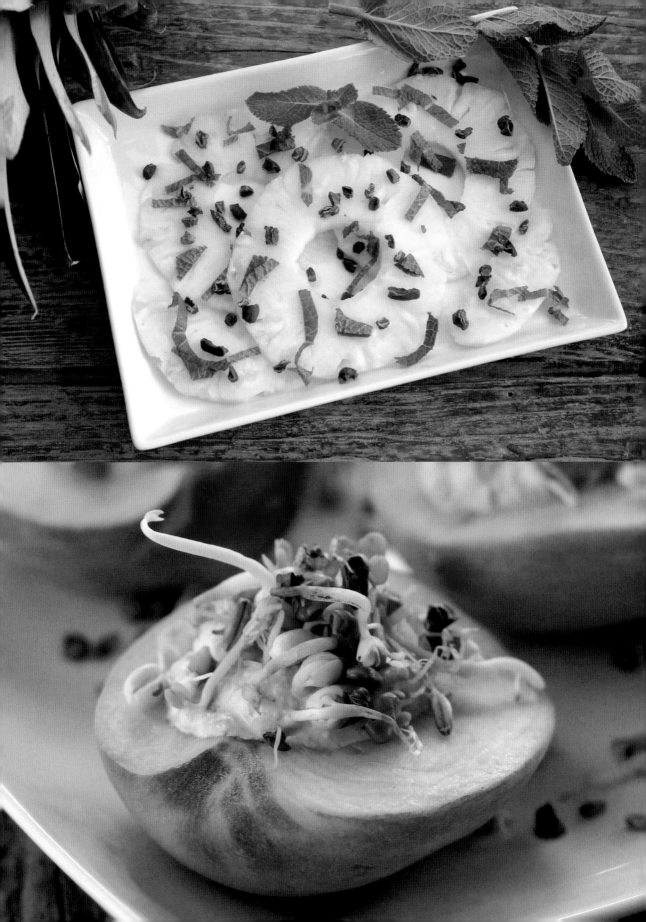

BANANA SPLIT

WITH COCOA NIBS AND GOJI BERRIES

SERVES 2
2 bananas
¼ cup (60 g) peanut
butter (see below)
2 tbsp (16 g) **cocoa nibs**
2 tbsp (15 g) **goji berries**

NUTRITIONAL VALUE
per portion

kcal	kJ	Protein	Fat	Carbo-hydrate
280	1,160	7	15	28

1. Peel the bananas and cut them in half lengthways. Spread the peanut butter over the cut sides. Sprinkle the cocoa nibs and goji berries evenly on top.

It is easy to make your own peanut butter without any additives. Blend the raw peanuts in a powerful food mixer at its highest setting until smooth and creamy. Stop a few times to push the mixture down from the sides of the mixer with a spoon. If necessary, add a small amount of groundnut oil.

CHOCOLATE MOUSSE

WITH AVOCADO

SERVES 2
1 ripe **avocado**
2 fresh or dried **dates**
2 tbsp (8 g) raw **cocoa powder**
7 tbsp (100 ml) almond milk
1 tbsp (8 g) **cocoa nibs**
raw **cocoa powder** for garnish

NUTRITIONAL VALUE
per portion

kcal	kJ	Protein	Fat	Carbo-hydrate
230	960	4	17	16

1. Cut the avocado in half lengthways; scoop out the pit and then the flesh. Remove the date pits.

2. Whizz the avocado flesh, dates, cocoa powder, and almond milk in a blender until smooth. Divide the mixture between two dessert dishes and garnish with cocoa nibs and some cocoa powder.

You can also replace the avocado with a banana. To make it sweeter, add one or two more dates or some coconut sugar—nut spread works well too.

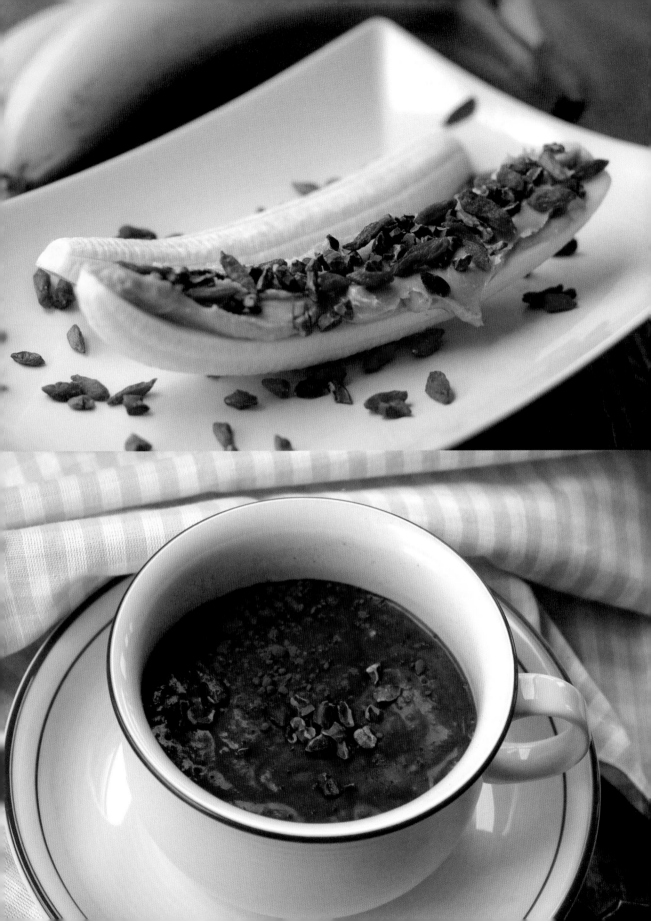

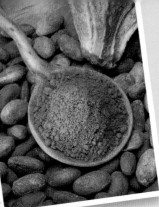

COCOA

Most of us think of "cocoa" as the familiar sweet chocolate drink made with milk. In its original form, however, it had a sharp, bitter taste: the indigenous people of Central and South America called it *xocolatl* (*xococ* meaning "bitter"; *atl* meaning "water"). They made the drink from crushed cocoa beans, water, chili, and vanilla. In 1544 the Spanish conquistador Hernán Cortés brought cocoa beans and the recipe for *xocolatl* home to the future King of Spain. In the 18th century the botanist Carl Linnaeus gave the cocoa tree the botanical name *Theobroma cacao*, which means "food of the gods," an indication of the esteem in which it was held by the Aztec. Raw cocoa contains magnesium, calcium, and dietary fiber as well as valuable antioxidants such as polyphenols and flavonoids. These substances keep the heart and circulation healthy and can prevent diseases such as heart attacks and strokes. They make blood vessels more elastic, lower blood pressure slightly, and are anti-inflammatory. Positive effects have also been demonstrated for our brains and responsiveness. Cocoa also contains the "happiness hormones" dopamine and serotonin: These are conducive to relaxation, reduced stress, and a greater sense of wellbeing.

Can cocoa and chocolate really be superfoods? Yes—though the valuable flavonoids in cocoa are destroyed when it is overheated or cow's milk is added. Traditional drinking powders made from cocoa and milk chocolate are normally heated to temperatures over 265 °F/130 °C and mostly contain more sugar than cocoa, not to mention milk powder and added flavorings, so these products are far from "clean." By contrast, healthy options include raw cocoa powder, dark chocolate with a high cocoa content, and cocoa nibs that have not been heated above 107 °F/42 °C. You can make clean and delicious drinking chocolate from raw cocoa powder and almond milk. So cocoa is an extremely beneficial foodstuff, if you choose unprocessed products and enjoy this scrummy but fat-rich pleasure in moderation. My own view is that, even if cocoa is healthiest in its raw state, I like to use it occasionally in baking—alternating cooked with raw cocoa fits nicely into my clean eating concept.

USES

My palate quickly adjusted to the relatively bitter taste of raw cocoa powder. I like to use it in smoothies, yogurt, chocolate mousse (p. 126), or in baking (walnut brownies, p. 130). Cocoa nibs (hulled cocoa beans broken into tiny chips) are great as a topping for breakfast dishes (overnight oats with chocolate and raspberry, p. 28) or desserts (pineapple carpaccio, p. 124; banana split, p. 126).

MACA

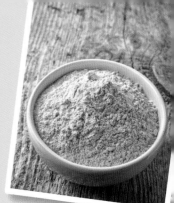

This superfood is native to the Peruvian Andes, where the yellow, red, or black roots of the maca plant (*Lepidium meyenii*) have been cultivated as a basic foodstuff and venerated as a healing plant for over two thousand years. The indigenous tribes in particular valued maca for its outstanding nutritional value and its powerful, energizing effect. This hardy plant adapted very well to the harsh climate of the high plateau: It withstands the wind, cold, severe variations in temperature, and high UV radiation. In a wider sense, the consumption of maca is said to increase our performance and resistance, to give us fresh energy to combat chronic fatigue, and to produce the mental balance we need to counteract stress.

Maca is still relatively unknown in Europe and North America, though demand has grown very rapidly in recent years. The aphrodisiac effect of "Peruvian ginseng" is increasing its popularity.

Its applications in natural medicine are extremely varied, however, as it is believed to: increase fertility, virility, and libido; regulate the hormonal balance; relieve the symptoms of menstruation and menopause; lower the cholesterol level; and boost the immune system and overall performance. As well as promoting muscle development, maca also increases mental focus. Metabolism and digestion are also improved. There have been many studies into the health benefits of long-term maca consumption, but the effectiveness of this healing plant has not yet been proved. What is undisputed, however, is the astonishingly high nutritional value of this bulbous tuber about the size of a radish. As well as all the essential amino acids, carbohydrates, valuable fatty acids, high-grade proteins, and sterols, the roots are also rich in vitamins, minerals, glucosinolates, and antioxidants.

USES

In Peru, the roots are mostly cooked or dried and made into a sweet porridge called "mazamorra." Maca is available in capsule form, as a liquid extract or powder, which is best suited to the clean eating concept. It tastes slightly earthy and bitter, yet it has a sweetish butterscotch flavor as well. It is not to everyone's taste, but the key to it is how it is prepared. Chocolate and vanilla notes work particularly well with it. To make a **hot maca** drink, simply heat a cup of cow's or plant-based milk and stir in 3 teaspoons of maca. If you like, you can add honey, agave syrup, or cinnamon. It makes a good caffeine-free substitute for morning coffee to kick-start the day. The powder is good for baking (p. 130), desserts and smoothies (pp. 18 and 20), or savory dishes (falafel, p. 80).

WALNUT BROWNIES

WITH MACA AND CAROB

MAKES approx. 8

⅔ cup (100 g) whole spelt flour
½ cup (50 g) raw **cocoa powder**
2 tbsp **carob powder**
1 tbsp **maca powder**
1 tsp (3 g) baking powder
salt
1 pinch vanilla powder or seeds
2 tbsp (30 g) butter
2 eggs
10 tbsp (150 g) soy or
other natural yogurt
5 tbsp (75 ml) honey
⅓ cup (35 g) shelled **walnuts**
some butter or oil for
the baking pan

NUTRITIONAL VALUE

per brownie

kcal	kJ	Protein	Fat	Carbo-hydrate
190	810	7	11	18

1. Pre-heat the oven to 355 °F (180 °C).

2. Sieve the flour into a bowl and mix in the cocoa, carob, maca, baking powder, salt, and vanilla.

3. 3. Add the butter, eggs, yogurt, and honey, and mix with a hand blender until smooth.

4. Coarsely chop the walnuts and stir them into the mixture. Grease a brownie pan (approx. 10 × 8 in / 26 × 20 cm), pour in the mixture, and smooth over the top with a spoon or scraper.

5. Bake on the middle oven shelf for about 25–30 minutes (see text box). Leave it to cool and then cut it into about eight pieces.

> Keep a close eye on the brownies toward the end of the cooking time. As they should be moist inside, some mixture should still be left on the skewer when you do a test (see p. 42). If you reheat the brownies just before you want to eat them, they taste even better.

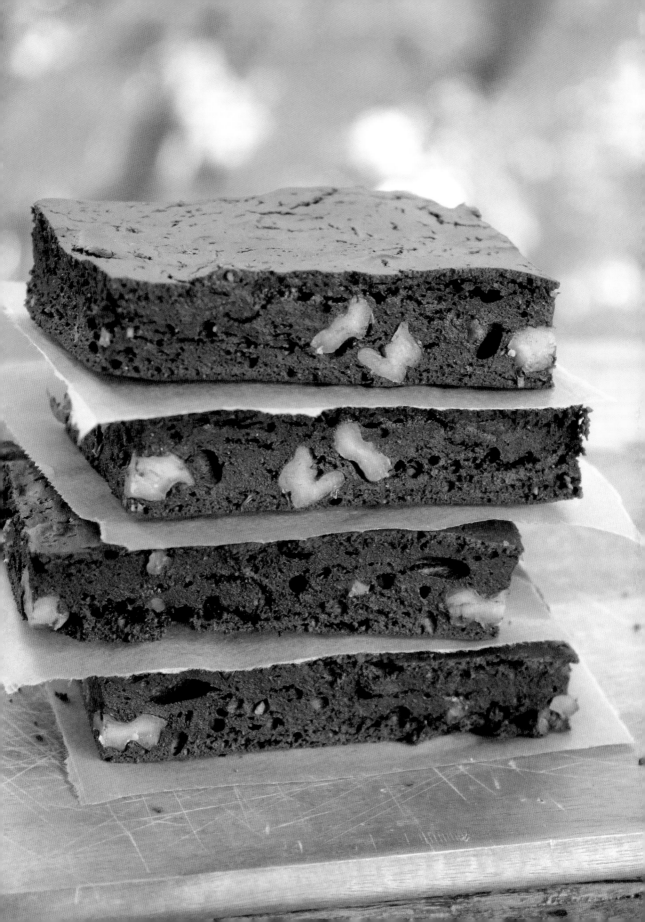

DATE PRALINES
WRAPPED IN GROUNDNUT CRUNCH

MAKES 5
100 g dried **dates,** pitted
¼ cup (20 g) rolled oat flakes
½ tsp (2 g) cinnamon powder
4 tbsp (20 g) unsweetened
cornflakes (100 percent maize)
¾ cup (100 g) unsalted
roasted groundnuts
3 tbsp (20 g) unsalted
roasted pistachios

NUTRITIONAL VALUE per date

kcal	kJ	Protein	Fat	Carbo-hydrate
250	1,030	8	14	24

1. Using a powerful food mixer, whizz together the dates, oat flakes, and cinnamon until smooth. Shape the mixture into five balls, adding some water if needed.

2. Whizz together the cornflakes, groundnuts, and pistachios. Divide the mixture into five portions and roll them out thinly. Place one date ball on top of each, and wrap the groundnut mix around them, using damp hands if necessary.

3. Put them on a plate in the refrigerator for 30 minutes, then serve.

> The pralines will keep in the refrigerator for at least a week. Instead of just wrapping the date pralines with the groundnut mix, you can also make two different types of praline.

CHOCOLATE STUFFED DATES

SERVES 2
8 dried or fresh **dates**
3 tbsp (40 g) cream cheese
2 tbsp (30 ml) agave
syrup or honey
1 tbsp (5 g) raw **cocoa powder**
1 tbsp (5 g) **carob powder**
2 tbsp (15 g) salted
pistachios, shelled
a few pistachio kernels to garnish

NUTRITIONAL VALUE per date

kcal	kJ	Protein	Fat	Carbo-hydrate
100	400	1	3	16

1. Cut the dates in half lengthways and remove the pits.

2. Combine the cream cheese, agave syrup, cocoa, and carob using a fork.

3. Add the very finely chopped pistachios, and mix well.

4. Stuff the dates with the chocolate cream. Garnish with pistachios.

> You can also use raw cocoa powder instead of carob powder.

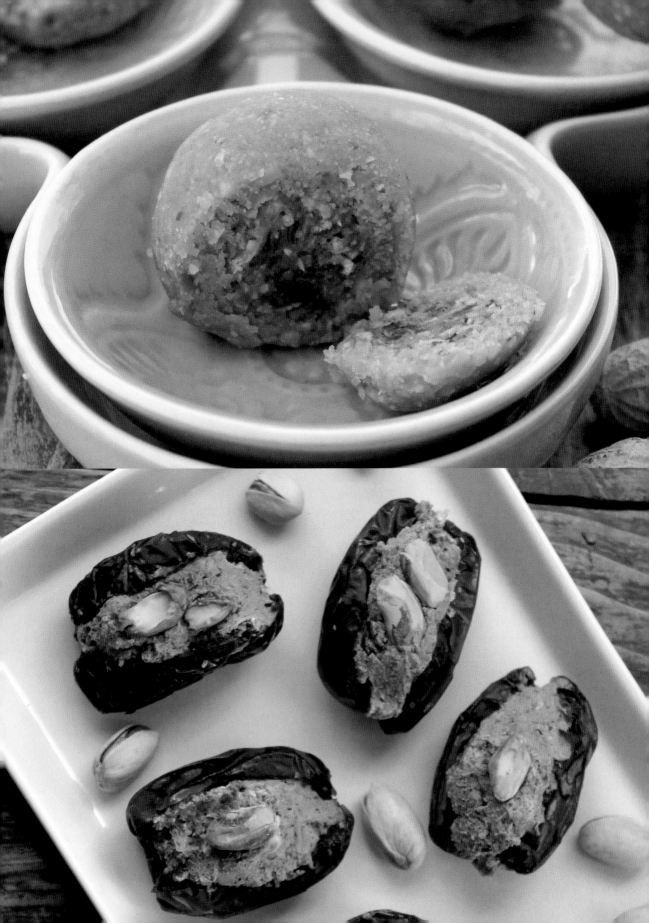

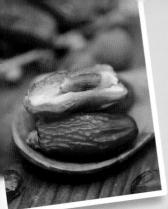

DATES

Known as the "bread of the desert," dates are a staple food for nomadic desert tribes. Date palms (*Phoenix dactylifera*) have been cultivated in their native lands—mainly Egypt, Pakistan, Saudi Arabia, and Iran—for over 5,000 years. Botanically, dates are classed as berries; there are believed to be as many as 1,500 varieties globally, differentiated by their color, in shades ranging from light to dark brown, through golden yellow to reddish. Their size, firmness of flesh, sugar content, and flavor can vary considerably.

Dried fruits are easy to transport and have a very long shelf life on account of their high natural sugar content (60–70 percent). Despite the high amount of fructose, dates are not fattening if eaten in moderation. In fact, they are a healthy alternative to sweets and ordinary sugar, as well as giving you a quick energy boost—one reason why sportsmen and women value this clean eating snack. Dates provide us with important minerals, which we tend to otherwise lose in part through sweat. This includes magnesium and potassium, which are good for the heart and muscles, and iron, folic acid, zinc, and lots of calcium.

Dates also contain vitamins A, B, C, and D. Potassium and B vitamins can reduce blood pressure, while the high level of dietary fiber stimulates the digestive system, staves off hunger pangs, and gives a prolonged feeling of fullness. Dates also have the amino acid tryptophane, which the body needs to produce melatonin. This so-called "sleep hormone" is effective in the treatment of nervous tension, anxiety, and sleep disorders.

USES

Common to all date varieties is their intensely sweet, caramel flavor. Dates are available fresh, dried, or frozen. I use my own homemade date paste as a natural sweetener, which is fine for the clean eating concept when used judiciously. To make it, simply pit 7 oz (200 g) of dates, and soak them in 7 tablespoons (100 ml) of water for 30 minutes. Then whizz them into a smooth paste using a mixer or blender, and spoon it into a screw-top jar. Kept in the refrigerator, the paste will stay fresh for at least a week. It adds an interesting dimension to desserts, baking, and drinks, as well as to savory dishes like salads or Asian food. I like to eat dates in their natural state as a snack between meals, as pralines wrapped in peanut crunch (p. 132) or in a salad with dates and pistachios (p. 72).

CAROB

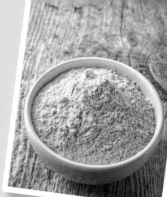

Carobs are the legumes (pods) of the carob tree (*Ceratonia siliqua*), which is widely cultivated in its native Mediterranean region and subtropical parts of other countries including the United States. It is also known as the "St John's Bread" tree—from the story in the Bible where John the Baptist sustains himself in the desert on carob. The chocolate-brown pods are harvested from August to October and ripen after being picked. In the growing regions they are eaten fresh or dried, either in their natural form or processed as a syrup, juice, or honey equivalent. Elsewhere, carob is available in powder form, made from the dried, ground, and partly roasted fruits. The nutritious pods also contain hard seeds, which are used to make carob gum—a practical, gluten-free thickening agent used in food production.

The powder is naturally sweet. Its fruity, caramel-like flavor makes a good substitute for cocoa in many recipes. Compared to standard processed cocoa powder, which contains milk powder and ordinary sugar, it is a healthy, lactose-free alternative (carob cocoa, see below). Unlike green or black tea, carob generally does not contain any stimulants like caffeine or theobromine, which also makes it suitable for children. Carob contains heaps of dietary fiber, which is good for the digestion, as well as proteins, vitamins A and B, calcium, and iron. It is rich in antioxidative polyphenols, which have a beneficial effect on the cardiovascular system in particular. In natural medicine, carob is also used to regulate the digestive system—effective in treating both constipation and diarrhea. Regular consumption of low-fat carob powder is also believed to lower blood fat levels and stimulate the fat burning process.

USES

The highest amount of healthy ingredients are found not in roasted dark brown cocoa powder, but in raw, light brown carob, which I use exclusively for this very reason. Though it has a unique taste, raw carob powder is similar to raw cocoa powder, only less bitter and tangy. Amounts of cocoa and carob powder in a recipe are directly interchangeable, spoon for spoon, though carob tastes far sweeter. Its high fructose content makes carob a popular natural sweetener. Carob gives desserts, cakes, and homemade nut milk and nut spread a different, distinctive flavor (walnut brownies, p. 130; and chocolate dates, p. 132). It can be used in marble cake, as well as in mousse, cream, ice cream, pudding, or drinks. To make carob cocoa, simply heat a cup of (plant-based) milk and stir in 1 teaspoon of carob powder.

QUINOA COOKIES
WITH CRANBERRIES

MAKES 6–8

6 tbsp (80 g) white **quinoa**
1 cup (150 g) whole spelt flour
3 tbsp (20 g) ground almonds
1 tsp (3 g) baking powder
salt
3½ tbsp (50 g) soft butter
1½ tbsp (20 g) raw cane sugar
⅔ cup (80 g) dried
unsweetened **cranberries**
⅔ cup (150 ml) almond milk

NUTRITIONAL VALUE

per cookie (for 8)

kcal	kJ	Protein	Fat	Carbo-hydrate
210	860	4	8	28

1. Rinse the quinoa well in a sieve under cold running water until it runs clear. Heat ⅔ cup (160 ml) of water in a pan and simmer the quinoa gently for 10 minutes, stirring occasionally. Drain and leave to cool.

2. Pre-heat the oven to 350 °F (175 °C).

3. Combine the quinoa in a bowl with the spelt flour, almonds, baking powder, and salt. Add the butter, sugar, cranberries, and almond milk. Knead well with the dough hook of a hand mixer.

4. Using your hands, shape the dough into six to eight flat cookies and place them on a baking pan lined with wax paper.

5. Bake the cookies on the middle oven shelf for about 20 minutes.

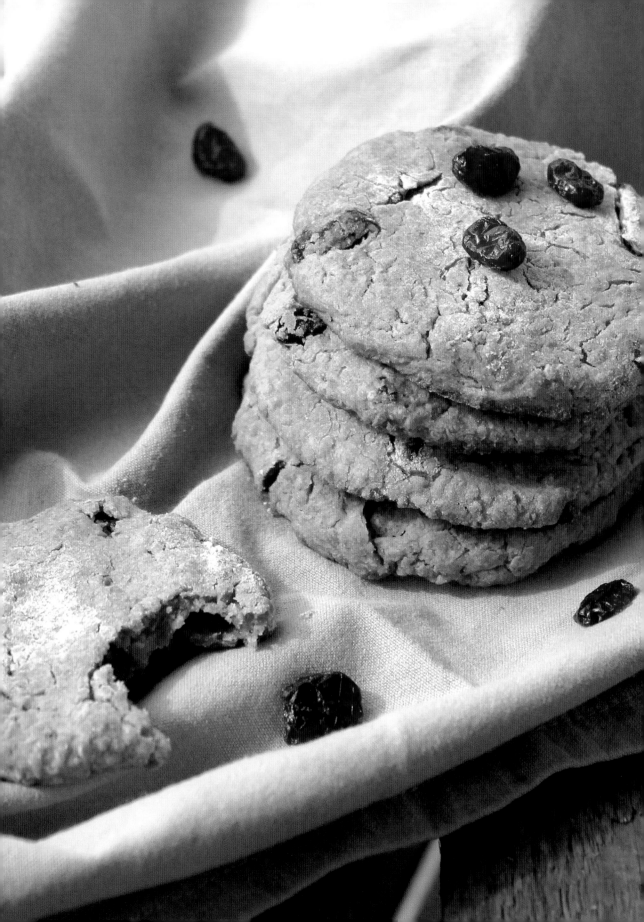

SUPERFRUIT SALAD

SERVES 2

3½ oz (100 g) **blueberries**
1 apple
½ pineapple
1 banana
1 kiwi
½ mango
3½ oz (100 g) strawberries
1 **lemon**
2 sprigs fresh mint
2 tbsp (16 g) **goji berries**

NUTRITIONAL VALUE

per portion

kcal	kJ	Protein	Fat	Carbo-hydrate
340	1,420	4	2	71

1. Wash and drain the blueberries. Wash the apple, remove the core and stem, and dice it.

2. Peel the pineapple. Cut off the hard inner core and brown "eyes." Finely dice the flesh.

3. Peel and dice the banana, kiwi, and mango. Wash the strawberries, remove the stems, and finely dice the flesh.

4. Squeeze the juice from the lemon and mix it through the superfruit salad along with the goji berries and washed, finely chopped mint leaves.

> The red "pearls" of a fresh pomegranate also make a wonderful addition to fruit salad. Mint and goji berries make it fresh and aromatic.

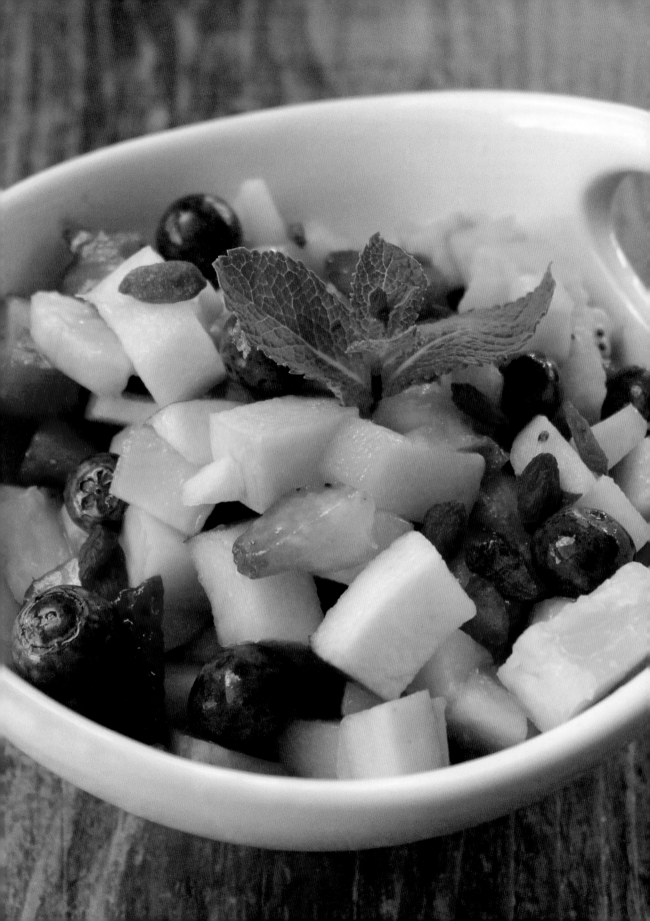

NUT PARCELS
WITH CHIA AND CRANBERRIES

SERVES 2

1¾ cups (225 g) whole rye flour

⅔ cup (150 g) chilled butter

3 tbsp (40 g) raw cane sugar

salt

1 egg

5 tbsp (45 g) almonds

5 tbsp (35 g) shelled **walnuts**

scant 2 tbsp (30 g) **chia seeds**

4 tbsp (30 g) dried
unsweetened **cranberries**

½ unwaxed **lemon**

½ cup (125 ml) milk

NUTRITIONAL VALUE

per portion

kcal	kJ	Protein	Fat	Carbo-hydrate
1400	5,860	27	98	102

1. Sieve the flour into a bowl. Cut the butter into small pieces and add it to the flour with the sugar, salt, and egg. Knead it into a smooth dough with your hands. Put plastic wrap around the dough and chill in the refrigerator for 1 hour.

2. Grind or blend the almonds, walnuts, and chia seeds finely and put them in a bowl. Coarsely chop the cranberries and add them too. Rinse the lemon in hot water and pat it dry. Grate the zest of half of the lemon and squeeze out the juice. Put the zest and juice in the bowl. Bring the milk to a boil, pour it into the bowl as well, and mix everything together with a wooden spoon. Leave the filling to soak for 15 minutes.

3. Roll out the dough between two sections of plastic wrap to make a square (approx. 1 in / 3 cm thick). Divide it into about 16 small squares.

4. Pre-heat the oven to 355 °F (180 °C).

5. Put 1 teaspoon of filling in the middle of each dough square. Fold two of the opposite corners into the middle, overlapping each other, and press them together carefully.

6. Place the nut parcels on a baking pan lined with wax paper. Bake on the middle oven shelf for about 15 minutes.

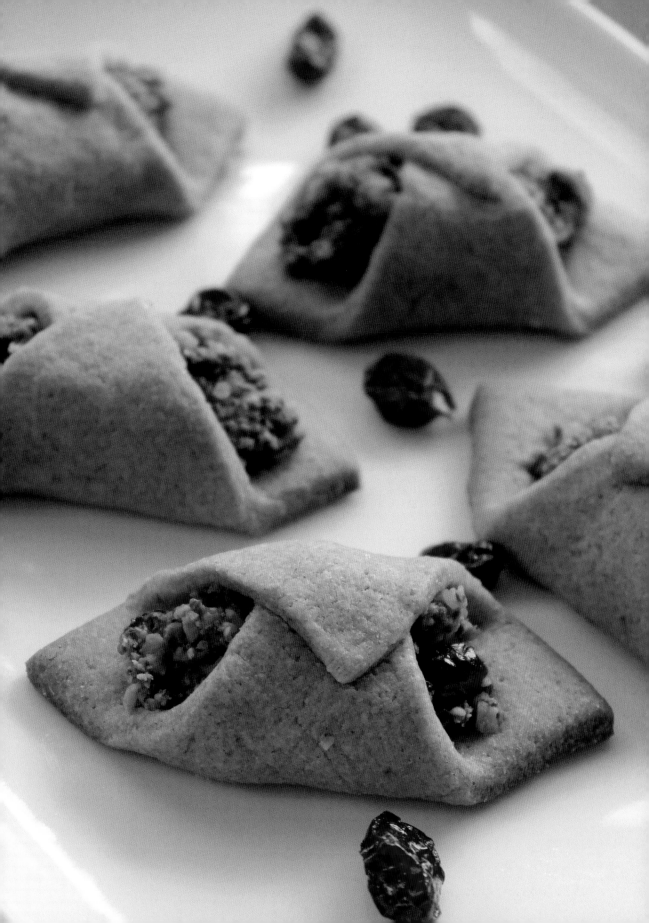

INDEX

SUPERFOOD PROFILES

Abbreviations and Quantities

1 oz = 1 ounce = 28 grams
1 lb = 1 pound = 16 ounces
1 cup = approx. 5–8 ounces* (see below)
1 cup = 8 fl uid ounces = 250 milliliters (liquids)
2 cups = 1 pint (liquids) = 15 milliliters (liquids)
8 pints = 4 quarts = 1 gallon (liquids)
1 g = 1 gram = 1/1000 kilogram = 5 ml (liquids)
1 kg = 1 kilogram = 1000 grams = 2¼ lb
1 l = 1 liter = 1000 milliliters (ml) = 1 quart
125 milliliters (ml) = approx. 8 tablespoons = ½ cup
1 tbsp = 1 level tablespoon = 15–20 g* (depending
    on density) = 15 milliliters (liquids)
1 tsp = 1 level teaspoon = 3–5 g * (depending
    on density) = 5 ml (liquids)

*The weight of dry ingredients varies significantly depending on the density factor, e.g. 1 cup of flour weighs less than 1 cup of butter. Quantities in ingredients have been rounded up or down for convenience, where appropriate. Metric conversions may therefore not correspond exactly. It is important to use either American or metric measurements within a recipe.

Picture credits

Photography: Hannah Frey, except p. 71: Stockfood, p. 36: Forest Starr & Kim Starr, flickr.com, p. 2, 17, 23: iStock, p. 16, 22, 33, 50, 55, 67, 76 84, 85, 107, 128, 134: Fotolia, cover: Shutterstock

© h.f.ullmann publishing GmbH
Original Title: *Clean Eating. Kochen mit Superfoods*

Author: Hannah Frey
Project management and editing of the original edition: Julia Genazino

Important information:
The contents of this book have been compiled to the best of the author's knowledge, and are based on meticulous research. They are not a substitute for expert medical advice. The suggestions in this book are provided without any guarantee or warranty on the part of the author or publisher, nor can they assume liability for any damage or harm caused by the advice given in this book.
This disclaimer applies in particular to the use and consumption of untreated raw milk and/or raw milk products, which the author and publisher strongly advise against due to the associated health risks. It is advisable not to serve dishes that contain raw eggs to very young children, pregnant women, elderly people, or to anyone weakened by serious illness. If in any doubt, consult your doctor. Be sure that all the eggs you use are as fresh as possible. Please note that bee pollen can be dangerous to those with allergies to bees, their products or other seasonal allergies.

© for this English edition: h.f.ullmann publishing GmbH
Translation from German: Ann Drummond in association with First Edition Translations Ltd, Cambridge, UK
Typesetting: Paul Barrett Book Production in association with First Edition Translations Ltd, Cambridge, UK
Layout: Satz- & Verlagsservice Ulrich Bogun, Berlin

Overall responsibility for production: h.f.ullmann publishing GmbH, Potsdam, Germany

Printed in Germany, 2016

ISBN 978-3-8480-1022-6

10 9 8 7 6 5 4 3 2 1
X IX VIII VII VI V IV III II I

www.ullmannmedien.com
info@ullmannmedien.com
facebook.com/ullmannmedien
twitter.com/ullmann_int

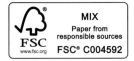